Contents

Health for a change

The provision of preventive health care in pregnancy and early childhood

Sue Dowling

CHILD POVERTY

in association with

First published by Child Poverty Action Group
1 Macklin Street, London WC2B 5NH
in association with the National Extension College, Cambridge

ISBN 0 903963 72 8

Any views expressed in this book are not necessarily those of CPAG

Cover photograph by Phil Coyne
Design by Hilary Arnott
Typeset by Enset
Printed by NEC Print

List of main projects described

Arbour, Liverpool
Ariel, Barnsley
Bermondsey Lamp Post
Child Care Switchboard Experiment, National Educational
   Research and Development Trust
Childminder courses. National Children's Centre, Huddersfield
Children's Centre, Thatcham
Children's Health Club, St Thomas' Community Health Council
Dial-A-Midwife Service, Shropshire
Dial-A-Midwife Service, West Berkshire
Early Visiting Scheme for families of Downs Syndrome babies,
   Southend-on-Sea
Educational Home Visiting: ILEA's south-east London scheme
Extended health visiting service: Barnet/Finchley
Extended health visiting service: Colchester
Extended health visiting service: Enfield
Extended health visiting service: Harrow
Family Care Line, National Children's Home, Manchester
Family Start, Oldham
Fundecker Playbus, National Children's Centre, Huddersfield
Geographical patch health visiting, Barnsley
Good Practices in Antenatal Health, National Council for
   Voluntary Organisations
Gypsy Health Project, Save the Children Fund
HELP, English-as-a-Second-Language Maternity Language Project,
   Leeds
Hampshire-Based Study Project
Health Visiting Crying Baby Scheme: Huddersfield
Health Visiting Crying Baby Scheme: Kingston and Richmond
Health Visiting Crying Baby Scheme: Plymouth
Health in Homerton
Home Aide Scheme, Social Services Department, Avon
Home-Start, Leicester
Homeless Family Scheme, Kensington, Chelsea and Westminster
Links with pregnancy testing agencies, Spastics Society (North-
   West Region)
Medical Social Work Project for Unsupported Parents, Bristol
Multi-Ethnic Women's Health Project, City and Hackney
Neighbourhood (patch) Based Services Project, Dinnington
Network, Watford
Newpin, Southwark

Open University Parent and Health Education Courses
Open-house child health clinic, Ore, Hastings
Organisations for Parents Under Stress (OPUS)
Park Cakes Ltd, Oldham: antenatal health promotion
Patients Committee, Aberdare Health Centre
Peckham Health Project
Postnatal support groups
Pre-School Organisations Committee (POC), Liverpool
School Concern Project, Community Service Volunteers
Scope, Southampton
Stillbirth Mutual-Aid Groups
Stockwell Health Project and the Mawbey Brough Health Centre
Strathleven Bonded Warehouses Ltd: antenatal health promotion
Street theatre health education, Blackburn
Thornhill Neighbourhood Project
Voluntary Service Co-ordinator, Milson Road Health Centre
Walk-in pregnancy clinic, Bolton
Workplace health education schemes, Trades Union Congress
Workplace health education schemes, Spastics Society

Abbreviations

AHA   area health authority
DHA   district health authority
DHSS   Department of Health and Social Services
GP   general practitioner
HA   health authority
HEC   Health Education Council
HV   health visitor
LEA   local education authority
NHS   National Health Service
OPCS   Office of Population Censuses and Surveys

Acknowledgements

Thanks must be given first to all the people who have provided the material for the study on which this book is based. Without their experience and ideas, it would not have been possible. Assistance was also given by the Royal College of General Practitioners and other relevant professional associations and colleges.

I owe much to many others, too. Ionna Burnell was the research assistant to the study and together with Jenny Whitfield and Lynne Harrison did much to establish it in its first year. The staff of the Department of Community Health, Bristol University, have provided me with continuous support. I am particularly grateful to Ralph Midwinter; also to the many secretaries who have given me so much practical assistance. Other members of the University to whom I am indebted for their advice are Charles Hannam and Michael Power.

The following people have allowed me to quote at some length from their work: Denise Hevey, Gwen Hiskins, Brian Jackson, Marion Walters and Linda Wonacott. I am most grateful for their generosity.

Thanks are also due to all those who have commented on and assisted in the production of the book as it has evolved through its several drafts. In particular I should mention Hilary Arnott, Jonathan Bradshaw, David Bull, Steve Burkeman, Jean Coussins, Maureen Fraser, Tom Heller, Chris Lyall Grant, Ros Morpeth, Helen Rosenthal, Alex Scott-Samuel, Roger Toulmin and Peter Townsend. I also gratefully acknowledge the assistance of CPAG and the DHSS who, respectively, sponsored and funded the study 'Ways of Reaching the Consumer in the Antenatal and Pre-School Child Health Services'. The book has been produced with the financial assistance of the DHSS and the Jack Tizard Memorial Fund, to whom many thanks.

My final thanks go back to the time, some ten years ago, when I was living and working in an inner city neighbourhood of East London. It was there that I received my grounding in community medicine. For this I owe much to local families, to a health visitor, Miss Theison and a paediatrician, the late Dr Ronnie MacKeith. From them I learnt the real meaning of the term 'inequality in health' and the difficulties of such communities in acquiring adequate health care when they need it. It was this experience, more than anything else, which prompted me to write this book.

Although so many people have encouraged and helped with this book, it is important to emphasise that the views expressed in it are my own. They are not necessarily those of the organisations and individuals associated with the study.

Foreword by the
Child Poverty Action Group

At the end of 1982, an all-time record of 7 million people — one in eight of the population — were dependent upon supplementary benefit. Unemployment, the biggest single cause of the dramatic increase in poverty since the late seventies, was still rising. The extent of the poverty which now exists will damage the life-chances of the next generation, as well as the present one.

Whilst campaigning for a coherent long-term government programme against poverty, based on the redistribution of income and wealth, CPAG also works to ensure that benefits services and opportunities which already exist are made available and are taken up by those who most need them. In the health field, good antenatal care and services which reach those who are particularly vulnerable to poverty and therefore to ill-health, can deliver a significant bodyblow to the recurrence of deprivation in successive generations and the pattern of severe inequalities in health which are endemic in our society and which government policies and administration, especially the NHS, have so far failed to break down.

In 1978 CPAG joined with the DHSS to organise a national conference: 'Reaching the Consumer in the Antenatal and Pre-school Child Health Services'. This study of innovative ways of reaching people with preventive health care during pregnancy and the early years of childhood has arisen from that conference. It is a contribution to the much wider debate which questions the scope and character of health services as well as their detailed organisation. Clearly, the two aspects cannot be shut off from one another in a clear-cut manner; indeed, many of the examples in this book will show how an organisational effort to reach a particular group of women effectively brings about change in the character of the service at the same time. An antenatal clinic in a shopping centre, for example, engages with women as healthy, normal equals, conducting their own lives; some hospital-based clinics, on the other hand, give women the impression they are patients suffering from a peculiar condition which requires them to be depersonalised and controlled.

The fact that this study is primarily a descriptive one, designed to inspire others to experiment with similar initiatives, should not detract from the underlying message: we should be looking for ways of removing the primary causes of inequality in health within our society so that the need for the predominently corrective strategies of the NHS is reduced. More resources must and can be found for poorer families.

The resources needed for health in pregnancy and early child-hood are of two types: first, to maintain and expand the NHS and the local authority services which influence health to meet the needs of the people. Initiatives from the voluntary sector should complement an adequately resourced statutory sector of health care, not compete with or threaten it. But secondly, a wider strategy has to be adopted in social and economic policies to redress structural inequalities. In particular, resources must be channelled urgently into the benefits system and welfare provision generally. Major relevant examples, which if neglected much longer may have grave repercussions for the health of the next generation, include the need for an adequate and inflation-proofed maternity grant, a child benefit which meets more of the true cost of a child, a return to a full schools meals service nationally and the extension of the long-term rate of supplementary benefit to the unemployed.

In CPAG's view, attention to the family income is vital if any long-term progress is genuinely desired in family health. As the Black Report concluded about our present inequalities in health: '. . . there is undoubtedly much which [can] be understood . . . only in terms of the more diffuse consequences of the class structure: poverty, working conditions, and deprivation in its various forms.'

CPAG is indebted to Dr Sue Dowling for undertaking this study and to the DHSS for providing most of the funding — to both we offer our thanks.

We would also like to express our gratitude to the Jack Tizard Memorial Fund for its generous donation towards the publication of this book. We hope that *Health for a change* will help to improve the life-chances of our children. This would be a fitting tribute to Jack Tizard.

Jean Coussins
July 1983

Introduction

Some thirty-five years after the founding of the National Health Service there is much evidence that we have failed to achieve one of its main objectives: *all* people should have equality of access to health care. The parents and young children who are most at risk from ill-health and premature death are still those for whom our preventive health services are least available and least used. They include the families of unskilled workers, those living in poverty, in depressed inner city neighbourhoods, the homeless and those whose first language is not English.

The main place for the NHS's preventive health service must be in the community, outside hospitals and other residential institutions. Governments have emphasised repeatedly that the health and social services should shift a greater proportion of their resources into this sector of care, particularly for children and other priority groups, such as the elderly (DHSS 1976c, 1981a, 1981c). Progress has been pitifully slow. The National Health Service looks more like a National Disease Service and the resources for promoting health in our health authorities are generally inadequate.

Although essential, an increase in resources is unlikely, by itself, to solve the problem of equality of access to preventive services. It is relatively easy to deliver health care to patients in hospital beds. In the community, people are less accessible. Here, the way in which care is provided may be particularly influential in determining whether families accept, ignore or reject it. Surprisingly little attention has been given to the research and development of different methods of health service delivery in the community. We seem to be concentrating on evaluating the nature of the actual care provided: how it can be improved and whether it is effective. These are vital questions. But it is equally important to study the processes which will ensure that this care reaches the people who need it.

This book is about this neglected area of study. It is based on a project which has attempted to map out new developments in the way preventive health care in pregnancy and early childhood is provided. It describes over sixty schemes in England and Wales, many of them probably unknown outside their immediate neighbourhood. The book is for those who plan, manage and deliver such services: health visitors, midwives, GPs, community physicians, administrators, clinical medical officers and community health councils, people working in local authority services, voluntary organisations and parents themselves. In addition, it seems likely that the study will be relevant to the people providing care for other groups in the community such as the elderly. Its findings point to the creativity and energy for change which exists within the NHS, as well as the other services concerned with health.

My focus on methods of health service delivery should not be interpreted as an affirmation that the NHS or the various health professions working in it can, on their own, solve the inequalities in health experience within our society. The conclusions of the Black Report (1980) show that such a view would be naive and untrue. National and local policies which are beyond the control of the NHS and which tackle the economic and social disadvantage of large numbers of parents and young children have a vital part to play. The concern of this book is that the contribution which *can* be made by preventive health services reaches all those who need it.

The study and how it was conducted

The aim of the study has been to identify ways of working which illustrate the processes involved in delivering preventive health care to all pregnant women and pre-school children: and particularly to those whom the health services find it difficult to reach.

To identify relevant schemes and collect information, letters were sent to every area health authority and community health council in England and Wales in the summer of 1979. The study was advertised as 'Ways of Reaching the Consumer in the Antenatal and Pre-School Child Health Services'. Over forty voluntary agencies, as well as numerous individuals such as teachers, social workers, pharmacists and trade union officials, were also contacted. Information was gathered from a wider audience by publicity in various medical, nursing, social work and educational journals, as well as in the national press.

Replies were received from 56 per cent of the health authorities and 42 per cent of the community health councils. In addition, some eighty individuals responded, representing the whole range of agencies contacted. The nature of the replies varied greatly. Some were short, saying they knew of no initiatives of the type sought. Others contained long lists of activities thought to be relevant. Descriptions ranged from a few words, 'health visitor liaises with childminders', 'toys and tea in antenatal clinic', to several pages of descriptive material. Most, however, were only a few lines or paragraphs long.

It was impossible to follow up all the schemes identified. The choice of those investigated further was influenced by factors such as their relative novelty and the ease with which more detailed descriptive material could be acquired. Gradually, by further probing through correspondence, telephone calls and in a few cases by visits, a picture was built up of the way in which many of these schemes worked, their success in reaching those they were aimed at and the way they had developed. It would be wrong to suggest, however, that this was an easy process or that it was successfully achieved in all cases. Those involved in the schemes were usually too busy with their everyday work to reflect on the way they were doing it or record the evidence of their success. Indeed, in planning the study, the time it takes to help projects and individuals develop this type of information was considerably underestimated. This may be an important observation for anyone setting out on a similar exercise.

Strenuous attempts were made to acquire objective measures of the scheme's successes when they were easily available: for instance, the numbers of people contacting a service before and after the introduction of a new way of working. However, such data depended on the presence of reliable records over several years. As these were not available in the majority of schemes, subjective assessments of their successes and problems were sought. Whenever possible these were recorded from several different sources.

Ultimately all this material was collated and written into case studies which were sent to the informants to check their accuracy and receive their comments. Errors of fact were then corrected and differences in interpretation were investigated further.

Examination of the material collected made it apparent that key concepts, such as *health, health services* and *consumer*, had to be clarified. The overall response of informants indicated that health in pregnancy and the early years of life was, indeed, seen as something which embraced social, economic, educational and psychological wellbeing, as well as physical health. It was seen as a state characterised by the absence of disease and disability and also by the achievement of a person's maximum potential in terms of their physical, intellectual, emotional and social development. It involved many agencies besides the NHS. In describing the findings of the study I have followed this wide interpretation of health and the services for health.

The nature of the material collected in the study also forced a re-interpretation of the phrase 'reaching the consumer'. The simplistic idea of an active service reaching out to a passive consumer had to be abandoned: several schemes showed parents and even children initiating and developing preventive health care schemes independently from or as equal partners with the professional providers.

The way the book is arranged

The volume of material collected in the study proved so great that it has been impossible to include it all in the book. In general, descriptions of projects and particular ways of working have been omitted only where one or two other almost identical examples are included.

In deciding how to arrange the material there has been the question of whether to describe schemes for pregnancy separately from those for pre-school children. For several reasons I have decided against this. Although the planning and management of NHS services for these groups are, on the whole, separate, there are many workers and agencies involved with providing preventive care both before and after birth: midwives, health visitors, GPs, social workers and some of those working in voluntary schemes. Many of the projects described do not see birth as a significant dividing line for their services: health in pregnancy is an integral part of health in childhood. It also seems that the processes involved in making contact with a local population of people with preventive health care — especially those whom the health services find most difficult to reach — are probably little different either before or after birth.

The chapters are arranged to reflect the major types of agencies providing preventive services for the health of pregnant women and pre-school children. Chapters 2 to 5 show how the NHS and health professionals are modifying their ways of working to make their services more available and attractive. Chapters 6 to 8 give examples of the special contribution which resources outside the NHS can make to the delivery of preventive health care for pregnancy and early childhood: the education services (chapter 6), the personal social services (chapter 7) and the voluntary sector (chapter 8). Chapter 9 outlines some practical ways in which all these different agencies are trying to overcome the many barriers which separate them so that they can work together to increase the availability of preventive health care for all families. Chapter 10 moves from the providers of services to the so-called 'consumers'. It describes how groups of parents and even children are beginning to modify and challenge factors which influence health in their neighbourhoods, including, of course, their local health services. The notes at the end of each chapter include the names and addresses of key contacts for each of the schemes described. It is hoped that this will enable readers to follow further any ideas or ways of working which seem relevant to their own area of work.

For readers wanting to identify the new district health authorities which correspond to area health authorities mentioned in the text, a word of explanation is needed. At the time when this study was carried out there were regional and area health authorities. Many of the latter were subdivided into smaller health districts. In April 1982, area health authorities were abolished and new district health authorities were created. Most of these district health authorities are smaller than the old area health authorities.

To find the new district health authorities which have replaced any area health authority mentioned in the text, readers are referred to the *Hospitals' Year Book 1982*, published by the Institute of Health Services Administrators. First, look up the area health authority concerned and identify its regional health authority. Then turn to the blue supplement pages of the *1982 Year Book*. These list the new district health authorities within each regional health authority, indicating, where possible, their relationship with their old area health authorities and health districts.

The study's limitations

When interpreting the findings of any study, it is important to appreciate the limitations imposed by its design. In the case of this study it may be useful to note these before proceeding to further chapters.

1. The sample of schemes described in the following pages is far from random. By design the study has produced a picture of the unusual — a glimpse of the fast-moving and innovatory fringe of antenatal and pre-school care which is not typical of these services as a whole.

2. The schemes described cannot give a complete picture of this field of innovation and service development. Readers will wonder why project x or y has not been included. Maybe they were not reported to the study or there was insufficient time or space to include them. Although there is no way of knowing the type of projects which were missed, it seems likely that these contained an excess of the smaller and more recently established ones which had not yet caught the attention of the authorities who were contacted for information. They may also have been those of which, for one reason or another, the informants did not approve. The way in which the final selection of schemes for inclusion in the book was made provided another route by which certain types of bias could have been introduced.

3. The picture presented in this book is like a snapshot representing an outline of developments occuring in one short time period in the early 1980s. The scene is constantly changing. By the time this book reaches the reader, some of the schemes will have changed, others will have disappeared, while new developments will have arisen.

4. The study is primarily descriptive. On the whole it has not been possible to evaluate objectively the success of the ways of working which are described. By design, the schemes included are those which seem to suggest useful insights into the processes involved in delivering services so they reach their target groups. Hopefully, these descriptions will provide starting-points for others to develop detailed evaluative studies of some of the types of schemes described.

5. This book offers no blueprints. What is appropriate in one situation may be misplaced in another. It is a learning resource, an 'ideas machine' for the planners, providers and consumers of health services. It points to the wealth of creativity and experience which exists within the services and among local communities. It may reveal clues about the most appropriate ways of managing and deploying our resources for health so that they reach those who need them most.

1 Background to the study

The children of today are the parents and providers of tomorrow. Even before their birth, their health or lack of it may affect the quality of life of future generations. The provision of health programmes which prevent disease and promote health in pregnancy and early childhood are consequently vital. This has been the conclusion of many major reports including the Court Report on Child Health (1976), The House of Commons Expenditure Committee on Preventive Medicine (1977), the Short Report on Perinatal Mortality (1980) and the Black Report on Inequalities in Health (1980).

Detailed reviews of our current knowledge about health in pregnancy and childhood are available elsewhere (see for instance Blaxter, M. 1981). Here I will point only to a few indicators of the persisting but changing need for preventive health care at these times.

At first sight, all looks well. Maternal deaths are now rare and stillbirth, perinatal and infant mortality rates[1] are low and continue to fall. The incidence of childhood deaths from infection has declined steeply since the start of the century. These changes are probably more due to improvements in families' nutrition, income, hygiene, housing and education than to medical treatment. Even conditions which have so far proved resistant to change, such as congenital malformations, are beginning to show signs of altering. For instance the introduction of genetic counselling and prenatal screening has been followed by a decline in the incidence of babies born with Down's Syndrome to older mothers and with abnormalities of the nervous system, such as spina bifida (Weatherall, J. 1982).

There seems a danger, however, that these improvements will lull us into a false sense of security. The moment of birth and the first months of life are still the most dangerous times of childhood. Seventy per cent of all childhood deaths are in the first year; 46 per cent occur in the first month (OPCS 1980). There are large geographical and social differences indicating that the factors causing premature death are unevenly spread and unevenly relieved. These inequalities are documented and discussed in detail in the Black Report (1980). Babies born to unskilled manual workers are twice as likely to die in their first year of life as babies born to professionals. The same scale of differences is found in children's later years of life. The causes of death which show the steepest social class gradients are those which are potentially preventable: deaths from accidents and respiratory infections. Low birth weight[2] is recognised as one of the most important adverse birth factors and has its highest incidence in social classes 4 and 5. The proportion of births which come within this birth-weight category has changed little in recent years. Such babies comprise only 7 per cent of all live and stillbirths, yet account for just over 55 per cent of all stillbirths and deaths in the first year of life (OPCS 1983d).

Though relatively few illnesses in the early stages of life now end in death, they may result in various degrees of discomfort, anxiety or disability and require medical attention. It is important not to lose sight of the Court Report's observation:

. . . the illusion exists that all childhood illness is diminishing. The facts are otherwise. There is a large amount of acute illness in children; some of it is minor, but much is severe and some life threatening or fatal.

Among the children of the 1970 British Birth Cohort (all children born between 5 and 11 April 1970), a quarter had an illness severe enough for admission to hospital for at least one night in their first five years of life.

Events which kill some foetuses and infants result in impaired development in others. The Warnock Report on Special Educational Needs (1978) estimated from various population studies that as many as one in six children are likely to require specialised and skilled help with their learning. This may be because of intellectual or educational retardation, psychiatric disorder or physical handicap. These problems are more common in children of unskilled manual workers and in those living in poor neighbourhoods than in their more advantaged peers. Many of these conditions are detectable early in life when there are opportunities to ameliorate or alter their impact on both the child and the family.

An important and related aspect of health in pregnancy or early childhood is the emotional and psychological wellbeing of parents, particularly mothers. Studies have shown that rates of depression in mothers with pre-school children are high, particularly in women of social classes 4 and 5 (Brown, G. and Harris, T. 1978). Depression at this time may impair a mother's ability to respond to the needs of her infant (Weissman, M. et al. 1972). It may result in manifestations of distress in the child (Rutter, M. 1966) as well as an increase in the incidence of accidents (Brown, G. and Davidson, S. 1978).

The tasks of prevention

Preventive health care operates at three levels. Primary prevention aims to prevent diseases and disabilities from ever occurring. Secondary prevention attempts to detect health problems as early as possible and then to treat and cure them. Tertiary prevention is concerned with established disease and disability and tries to minimise their impact and further complications.

The task of preventive health care in pregnancy and early life is to meet the various health needs of families at each of these three levels. The following paragraphs give a few examples of these health needs: the list is not meant to be comprehensive.

Medical

Examples include the occurrence of dangerous infectious diseases in pregnancy (e.g. rubella) and early childhood (e.g. polio, diphtheria, whooping-cough). These can be prevented primarily by immunisation. Potentially harmful conditions, such as anaemia and pre-eclampsia in pregnancy, and congenital dislocation of the hip and squints in early childhood, should be detected as soon as possible and treated. Established and incurable conditions such as some forms of kidney disease in pregnancy and cerebral palsy in early childhood also need to be identified early so that their complications can be minimised.

Economic and social

Poverty is on the increase. By the end of 1982, the number of people in Britain dependent on supplementary benefit reached a record level of seven million (House of Commons Hansard 1983b). An estimated 1.9 million children — roughly one child in every seven — will be living in such families in the year 1983/4 (House of Commons Hansard 1983a). This is twice as many as in the late seventies. Unemployment, the cause of this increase, continues to rise.

The numbers are larger when you take account also of families not receiving supplementary benefit. In 1979 (the latest year at the time of writing that official statistics have been published) there were approximately 4 million households containing some 6.1 million people living on or below the supplementary benefit level. They included nearly 1 million children. If families with incomes marginally above supplementary benefit are added, this figures rises to more than 2 million.

This growth in family poverty in large sections of society is likely to have serious consequences for the health of children. The Black Report (1980) concluded that the material deprivation associated with poverty is an important contributor to the greatly increased risk of death and ill-health in children of social classes 4 and 5 compared with those of social classes 1 and 2. For instance, accidents account for about a third of all deaths of children aged 1 to 14 years and shows a steep social class gradient. Children in the unskilled manual classes tend to live in more hazardous environments than their more advantaged peers, with cheaper and less safe forms of heating and less opportunity for supervised play in danger-free areas. Low income and its associated stresses are also linked to an increased risk of parental ill-health which, in turn, is likely to impair parents' ability to look after the safety and health of their children.

The social support of parents in looking after young children is also relevant to family health. Recent trends suggest that the availability of such support during pregnancy and childrearing may be decreasing for some parents. The proportion of families with dependent children headed by a lone parent increased from 8 per cent in 1972 to 12 per cent in 1980. The largest increase in the 1970s was among families headed by a divorced mother (OPCS 1982a). The proportion of all births which were illegitimate increased from 7 per cent in 1964 to 13 per cent in 1981 (Werner, B. 1982). The reduction in family size in the last few decades means that there are now fewer relatives to supports parents with young children. There are also signs that in urban areas, particularly inner city neighbourhoods and ethnic minority communities, families may be isolated by their fear of neighbours and also of people in positions of authority (Scarman, Lord 1981; Knight, B. and Hayes, R. 1981).

These types of social stresses may have a direct effect on the health of pregnant women and young children. Haggarty (1980) has pointed to the association between upsetting and stressful life events and an increase in vulnerability to infections in children. Brown and Harris's study (1978) of depression in women with pre-school children has shown its association with adverse life events characterised by loss and disappointment.

Educational

Parents need information with which to make important decisions about medical care and other factors which affect health, such as income maintenance, nutrition, smoking and drinking. Cartwright (1979) showed that among mothers having their first babies, those in social classes 4 and 5 were the least likely to feel that they knew enough about childbearing and rearing before they had their baby. They were also the group most likely to say that they would like to have known more. Yet these were the women least likely to go to antenatal preparation classes or to get their information from professionals.

Children have educational health needs too. The Headstart programme in North America has shown the positive impact which carefully designed and supported pre-school educational programmes can have on intellectual development in the early years of life (Lazar, F. *et al*. 1977).

Environmental

These include the need for pollutant-free air, food and water. Though the introduction of the Clean Air Act (1956) has done much to control industrial and domestic smoke emissions, other pollutants such as organic lead are increasing in the environment and may have a harmful effect on child development and health (Gloag, D. 1983). Cigarette smoking is another source of air pollution and is a major contributor to the incidence of low birthweight (Butler, N. and Alberman, E. 1969) and a cause of respiratory infections in children (Colley, J. and Reid, D. 1970).

In the last decade, in the general population, the proportion of women who smoke in the unskilled manual socio-economic group has changed little, while that in the non-manual and skilled socio-economic groups has declined (OPCS 1983b).

The providers of preventive health care

It follows from this classification of health needs in pregnancy and early childhood that preventive health care should involve medical, economic, social, educational and environmental strategies. It must therefore be the concern of society at many different levels: central government departments, local authority departments, health authorities, employers, trade unions, the voluntary sector of care and many other organisations as well as parents and children themselves.

The NHS therefore is only one part — albeit an important one — of a spectrum of agencies concerned with preventive care. The NHS provides most of this care for pregnant women in hospital antenatal clinics and classes staffed primarily by obstetricians and midwives. Antenatal care is also carried out in the community by GPs, community midwives and health visitors. In contrast, the majority of the NHS's childhood preventive care is community based: in general practices, in health authority child health clinics and in families' homes. Some of the key health professionals concerned include health visitors, GPs, clinical medical officers and hospital-based staff such as paediatricians.

Problems in delivering preventive health care

Research evidence has been reviewed elsewhere showing that the parents and young children with the greatest risks of premature death, disability and disease are those who are least likely to receive the NHS's preventive services in pregnancy and childhood (Blaxter, M. 1981; Townsend, P. and Davidson, N. 1982). A similar situation applies in many other services which may affect people's health at these times: for instance adult education and pre-school day care services (Dowling, S. 1978).

Research is now beginning to unravel the many factors which may be associated with these failures in use and delivery of services. We have known for a long time that the so-called 'poor users' of antenatal and child health clinics tend to be of a lower social class, living in poorer quality housing with lower educational qualifications than the parents who attend these services (Douglas, J. and Blomfield, J. 1958; Davie, R. et al. 1972). The former group may not have the necessary information about when and how to use the preventive health services. They may also have difficulties of transport and of meeting the financial costs of attending clinics regularly.

But as well as the 'poor users' we have to consider the concept of 'poor providers'. It is known, for instance, that the geographical distribution of health service resources tends to be mismatched with the need for them (Noyce, J. et al. 1974; West, R. and Lowe, C. 1976). Considering the health care provided, it is apparent that the way it is organised and delivered can be a major determinant of its availability for parents and children. For example, surveys of general practice have shown that health care staff may be difficult to contact when patients telephone after surgery hours, this problem sometimes being associated with the use of deputising services (Acheson Report 1981). In hospital antenatal clinics it seems that if the staff's work is centred on a particular task, such as taking blood pressures, examining urines or abdomens, rather than being focused on the pregnant woman as a whole, the experience and attitudes of clinic users to their health care may be adversely affected (Graham, H. and McKee, L. 1980). The dissatisfaction which women have expressed with their clinic visits (Garcia, J. 1982) may also relate to the size of the clinic staff's workload. Careful analysis may show that this is not always appropriate and may often be unnecessarily great (Hall, M. et al. 1980). This may make it difficult for staff to provide a more acceptable and attractive form of care.

The search for solutions

These then are a few of the problems known to be associated with the use and delivery of preventive health care programmes. But what type of changes will be effective in remedying them and how can these changes be introduced? One way of finding solutions to these questions is by means of action-research. Such projects may establish 'ideal' antenatal or child health preventive services in the community and monitor the way in which they work and their impact on health (for instance, the Easterhouse antenatal scheme in Scotland[3], the Thomas Coram Child Health Project in London[4], and the Riverside Child Health scheme in Newcastle[5]).

A somewhat different approach to the search for solutions is to recognise that within the context of the everyday work of health professionals, they often experiment with new methods of delivering preventive health services. It is important not to overlook these variations within our existing services: they are a rich source of ideas and spontaneous innovations suggesting how resources may be redefined and used in new and imaginative ways. Such ways of working are rarely thought of as 'experiments' in the research sense of the word. They are carried out, often with no special budget or staff, by the fieldworkers and managers who provide the day-to-day statutory and voluntary services in the district. Sometimes these experiments are the result of a conscious decision to change the nature of the services delivered. They may also be part of a more spontaneous and unconscious process: people are often surprised to be told that their method of providing health care is unusual or interesting.

The study of these types of innovations within our services is fraught with problems. They often lack clearly defined objectives, they cannot be controlled (in the research sense of that word) and they are difficult to evaluate, analyse and assess. Perhaps for these reasons they are rarely recorded or afforded space in the prestigious scientific journals which inform health professionals and policy-makers and managers of services. But they have advantages:

— they are cheap
— they are realistic, in the sense that they are occuring in the normal service environment with no special staff and resources
— they recognise the 'good' in the everyday services and thus may increase staff morale and perhaps even change patterns of work
— they provide an enormous variety of approaches, containing the originality, ideas and responses of hundreds of different people who are close to the needs of parents, children and the service providers.

The NHS has been criticised for being slow to introduce new ideas into health care organisation and delivery (Ham, C. and McMahon, L. 1982; Hunter, D. 1983). If its organisation is to evolve and adapt to the changing problems which we face it is important that the creative experiments in service delivery which are developing in our midst are identified. They should be recorded and, wherever feasible, evaluated. Information about these innovations should be disseminated widely so that the people shaping and running the services for health in each district can learn from the experience of others. This book attempts to map out some of the new developments in the delivery of preventive health care in pregnancy and early childhood and to disseminate information about them. It has been prepared in the belief that information is an important catalyst for change.

Notes

1 *Stillbirths:* late foetal deaths after 28 completed weeks of gestation. Rate expressed per 1,000 live and still births. *Perinatal deaths:* still births and deaths in the first week of life. Rates expressed per 1,000 live and still births. *Neonatal deaths:* deaths in the first 28 days of life. Rates expressed per 1,000 live births. *Infant deaths:* deaths at ages under 1 year. Rates expressed per 1,000 live births.
2 Defined as babies weighing less than 2,500 g.
3 Easterhouse Clinic Project, Social Paediatric and Obstetric Unit, 64 Oakfield Avenue, Glasgow G12 8LS
4 Thomas Coram Child Health Project, Community Paediatric Research Unit, St Mary's Hospital Medical School, London NW5 5RN
5 Riverside Child Health Project, Atkinson Road Infant School, Atkinson Road, Newcastle NE4 BXT

2 Parents and children – who and where are they?

It is recommended that the preventive health services for pregnancy and early childhood should make early and regular contact with every pregnant woman and every pre-school child (Maternity Services Advisory Committee 1982; Committee on Child Health Services 1976). Through these contacts appropriate health surveillance, care and information may be given.

If the maternity and child health services are to achieve these objectives, and plan their services appropriately, they must be able to locate all pregnant women and pre-school children. The complexity of this task should not be underestimated. In any health authority these populations are constantly changing. The parents and children most in need of health care are often to be found among those who frequently change their address or are 'invisible' to the health service for other reasons, such as homelessness.

This chapter focuses on four of the difficulties concerned with the accuracy of information needed to contact parents and children, and describes schemes which are trying to overcome these in the following ways:

— by identifying, as soon as possible, new parents and babies moving into populations, who need maternity and child health services
— by creating population registers which can quickly identify those whom the services have failed to reach
— by improving the accuracy with which surnames are recorded (people's main identifying features)
— by keeping contact with the families who are 'invisible' to the health services, because, for instance, they have changed their address or become homeless.

Identifying new members of the target population

The identification of the group of newly born children and their parents with whom the pre-school health services should be in contact (the 'target population') is relatively simple. Their names and addresses are available from statutory birth notifications (see page 18). For the maternity services, however, there is no equivalent method of identifying newly pregnant women, for example, by reference to their positive pregnancy tests. This section will therefore examine tried ways of identifying women as early as possible after their pregnancy has been confirmed, so that appropriate information and care may be offered.

In this task it is essential to remember that the beginning of a pregnancy can be an intensely private affair which women may be reluctant to communicate to outsiders, particularly if the pregnancy is not welcomed. The health service should move with sensitivity. There is a delicate balance between the rights of the community to health protection through an efficient health service and the rights of individuals to privacy.

Nevertheless, while recognising that rights of parents are important, the health service must try to ensure that at the point when a woman's pregnancy is confirmed, she is offered information which enables her to make appropriate decisions about her and her new baby's health and care. She should also be given the opportunity of contacting and linking in with the NHS maternity services, there and then (for evidence that this may not happen see Garcia, J. and Oakley, A. 1982).

Links with pregnancy testing agencies

Pregnancy testing is the first and sometimes the only chance for the health service to identify the names and addresses of pregnant women. There are now many different agencies which offer pregnancy testing. For instance, within health authorities there are hospital and family planning clinics. Also within the NHS, but independent from the health authorities, there are the GP services. Outside the NHS there are private services, such as pregnancy advisory bureaux. Pharmacists may also carry out the tests on their own premises or sell women pregnancy testing kits which they can use at home. The links between health authorities' antenatal services (clinics, obstetricians, midwives and health visitors) and the pregnancy testing services offered by GPs and the private commercial sectors often seem poorly defined, if they exist at all. The impression from this study is that they depend more on the goodwill of the staff concerned than on the structure of the health service.

Contact between GPs and health authorities' antenatal services appears to vary according to whether the GP offers his or her own antenatal services and, if so, the degree of sharing and co-operation between the two services. Some health authorities described how GPs pass the results of all positive pregnancy tests to the community midwives and health visitors, who then make sure the parents are offered antenatal care. Others said that their community midwives visit all the GPs' surgeries in their area to obtain these details. Some midwives clearly have considerable difficulties

from the medical records of the practice or from the files of the family practitioner committee. Many of these registers are computerised and are used, like the health authority registers, to identify children eligible for relevant preventive health programmes.

In addition, a few family practitioner committees (e.g. in Avon, Calderdale and Trent) are computerising the basic information concerning the patients of all the general practices in their area. This information can then be supplied to any GP who needs information on his/her practice population.

It is important to note, however, that all these GP registers include only those children who are registered with a general practice. Because parents may delay in registering their newborn child, GPs. age/sex registers are particularly incomplete for children in the first year of life (Fraser, R. and Clayton, D. 1981; Fraser R. 1982). Such inaccuracies may make them unacceptably imprecise for this vulnerable age group.

Improving the accuracy of recording surnames

Records, whether held on a computer or in a filing-cabinet, are only as accurate as the information which is written on them. People's surnames are their main identifying features on information systems — for instance, on their health service records or on population registers. Incorrect recording may result in them being untraceable within these systems. It can also lead to delays in finding notes, confusion between different sets of notes and irritation on all sides.

Asian surnames

A particular aspect of this accuracy problem has been highlighted by health workers in areas with large numbers of births to Asian parents. These workers tend to be familiar only with the British naming system, which places the common family name last in a person's order of names. Among the Asian communities there are several different naming systems. Muslims, for instance, traditionally use no common family name. Sikhs, though they usually have a family name, prefer not to give it for religious reasons. Instead, they may identify themselves by their religious names — Singh for men and Kaur for women (Henley, A. 1979).

A teaching programme for NHS staff Materials are now available to teach health service staff how to use the different Asian naming systems correctly and acceptably. These materials have been developed as part of a three-year project 'Asians in Britain' which is financed by the DHSS and King's Fund.[2] The teaching pack[3] is designed primarily for those who train record clerks, receptionists and nurses in the NHS. It contains a trainer's manual, a set of trainer's lecture notes, overhead projector transparencies, information booklets for the trainees, job-aid cards for trainees to use at work and a cassette giving the correct pronunciation for common Asian names. A modified version of the teaching material is available for GPs and their receptionists to study on their own if they cannot attend a full training session.

Keeping contact with 'invisible' families

The nature of population registers composed from birth notifications and GP records has been described above. Both these types of information system, however, may be inaccurate. Inaccuracies of address are probably more common than those of surname and may result in a considerable number of parents and young children becoming untraceable (Heward, J. and Clayton, D. 1980).

Incorrect addresses usually occur because the parents and/or child move home some time after their initial entry on the register. A national study of children born in 1970 showed that 57 per cent had moved at least once between birth and five years. Eleven per cent had moved twice, and another 11 per cent had moved three or more times (Butler N. *et al.*, forthcoming). Unless parents tell the NHS of their move, it is unlikely that the NHS will know their whereabouts until they sign on with a new GP or make themselves known at a hospital or health authority clinic. There may be long delays before this is done.

Recent reports have drawn attention to the considerable number of people in inner city areas who are not registered with a GP and the difficulties of some of them being accepted on to GPs' lists (London Health Planning Consortium: Primary Care Study Group, 1981, para 3.2; Leicester CHAR 1982). This may be because of the neighbourhood in which they live or because they are unpopular patients — for instance, the homeless and gypsies. Many such parents and young children may always remain 'invisible' to GPs, despite their need for health care.

Making contact with these families often depends on the community skills and knowledge of health visitors and community midwives and on their links with other neighbourhood workers. Such people are the eyes and ears of the health service. A health worker in an inner city area described her concern about the adolescents who were leaving home, but with nowhere to live and little income. Some of them were sleeping in derelict boarded-up buildings, others in the heating spaces at the top of tower blocks in the neighbourhood. A few of the girls were pregnant. Knowing their suspicion of people in authority, the health worker appreciated that contact with the antenatal services had to be introduced and made in a most sensitive manner.

The availability of such local knowledge seems to be related to the considerable trust and acceptance which health visitors, community midwives and others can establish within their communities. Aspects of their particular work situations which they described as contributing to this trust are:

— 'visibility' and availability on the streets, in the shops, launderettes, schools and playgrounds;
— length of time they have been in the neighbourhood: the longer the better
— size of the area in which they work: it should not be large
— involvement with the total community, not just those on the list of a GP or attending some other service agency (see chap. 9 for a discussion of geographical and health visitors attached to GPs)
— involvement in a wide range of local activities, not just those identified as a health concern.

Liaison health visitor posts

Liaison health visitor posts have been created in some health authorities for working with the staff and children's families on antenatal, postnatal and paediatric wards and the casualty departments of hospitals. Working across these different parts of the maternity and child health services, such health visitors are in a key position to identify and notify the authority of changes in children's circumstances and addresses.[4] They may also make contact with many families who, being unregistered with a GP, use the hospital casualty department for their primary care. In these circumstances they can tell the parents about the importance of having a GP and assist them in registering. They may also introduce them to their local health visitor and, if they are pregnant and receiving no care, link them with the maternity care staff.

Kensington/Chelsea/Westminster Homeless Family Scheme In Kensington and Chelsea and Westminster AHA a special scheme[5] was established in 1975 to link the health service with the various local authority housing departments who were placing homeless families in temporary accommodation within the authority's boundaries. A survey of all such families carried out by health visitors showed that large numbers were being placed by outside boroughs in bed-and-breakfast hotels. To quote a report of the survey:

Very rarely did the placing Authority notify the host Authority of the family placement, which became known to the health visitor or social worker only when the family presented itself at the Child Health Clinic or asked for a Day Nursery vacancy. Many of these families produced an enormous number of social problems resulting from their homelessness but had no social work support from the placing authority . . .

Statistics for the health authority show that the total number of homeless families in temporary accommodation has been steadily growing, with an increase in such families needing antenatal care. At the end of the first quarter of 1980, there were 612 families resident in temporary accommodation. These families included 180 mothers needing antenatal care, 301 children under 5 years and 154 children over 5 years. It was estimated that many of these families would have moved again within two or three months.

To try to ensure that such families received the health care they needed, the Area Nurse (local authority liaison) held regular meetings with the housing and social service departments of the main placing boroughs. Several initiatives developed. All the temporary accommodation used was vetted by environmental health officers for its suitability. The hoteliers were encouraged to make arrangements with local GPs for the emergency care of any person residing with them. In addition, the homeless family units were issued with street lists of the health authority, giving the addresses of all the child health clinics where health visitors could be contacted. Some of the units issued homeless families with an information sheet, stating the address and telephone number of the clinic nearest to their hotel or bed-and-breakfast accommodation.

The success and difficulties of this scheme have not been formally evaluated. From the comments of the senior nursing managers, however, it appears that it has considerably increased the contact of the health service with homeless families as they move through the authority. It should be noted, however, that at the start of the scheme the uncovering of this unknown and transient population, with their demanding health and social needs, greatly increased local health visitors' workload. This caused considerable difficulties until the number of health visitors employed was increased in the authority.

At the time of writing it is uncertain whether this scheme will continue. Three separate DHAs have now replaced the old single AHA — a reorganisation of services which seems to have made liaison with local authority departments difficult.

Links with voluntary groups

Network, Watford Network[6] is an example of a voluntary project which is working closely with health professionals in the community. It was started in 1975 by a community worker in the social services department to provide a network of people who act as street contacts for families. The job of these volunteers is to look out for and get in touch with any parent who moves into their street or anyone living there who has a new baby. They tell them about the facilities for young children in the area — including clinics and the health visiting services — and may offer to introduce them to other families in the street.

To establish the project the community worker set up a steering committee consisting of mothers, a health visitor, a pre-school playgroup advisor and herself. Together they developed a small network of street contacts covering a geographical area which contained about twenty-four roads. They found several people to act as the co-ordinators of the scheme in this area. These co-ordinators recruited, supported and kept in touch with the street contacts living in each of the roads. They also found out about local facilities for parents and young children and produced details of these in a 'resource pack'. These were given to each of the street contacts together with a Network sign for display in their windows.

From this small beginning Network has gradually grown into an organisation of over 300 street contacts and many neighbourhood and area co-ordinators covering much of the town and its surrounding area. The original steering committee has been expanded into a co-ordinating committee with the function of deciding the policy of Network and acting as an information exchange for all the different people working in it. A quarterly newsletter is produced and sent to all co-ordinators and street contacts.

So far there has been no formal evaluation of the different aspects of Network's work. However, the impression gained from talking with members of the co-ordinating committee and health visitors is that in some neighbourhoods it is succeeding in keeping in contact with many of the parents with young children. Health visitors commented that through Network they are sometimes alerted to families and health needs about which they were previously unaware.

When asked about problems, some of the volunteers in Network admitted that the organisation's middle-class image may be a disadvantage in gaining acceptance in some of the town's council estates. There also seems a consensus that Network's organisation may have become too complex and centralised. It is now felt that its main administration, policy-making and development should return to small neighbourhood or area units. To quote one of Network's voluntary officers:

> We've learned by hard experience that what works in one group of streets won't work in another. It's useful to have ways of

exchanging information and ideas between all the neighbourhoods — but beyond that a central hub of organisation may be
counter-productive. We seem to have distanced ourselves from
families by all our administration. Just tell anyone who's
thinking of starting something similar — keep it small and very
local. That's its strength.

In conclusion

The schemes described in this chapter are intended to improve the
completeness and accuracy of information needed to contact
parents and children during pregnancy and early childhood.
However the complexities of making and keeping contact with
these constantly changing populations should not be underestimated. Many of the schemes described depend on adequate liaison
— which in turn depends on trust — between the different agencies
working with families: for instance health workers and local
authority housing departments and voluntary organisations.
Most importantly they rely on the willingness of parents to divulge
information to people in authority in these services and their
understanding that this will only be passed to others with their
consent.

There is a delicate balance between the rights of the community
to health protection through an efficient health service and the
rights of each parent and child to privacy. At the time of writing
the Data Protection and the Police and Criminal Evidence Bills are
passing through the House of Commons. They contain clauses
which may seriously undermine the trust of parents and health
professionals in the security of the information needed for health
care. State intrusion into these sensitive areas of confidentiality
may deter some people from seeking medical assistance: for
instance those who live in inner city neighbourhoods where there
may be a distrust of authority and the police. These are the very
parents and children who tend to have the greatest need for our
maternity and child health services. Therefore it is imperative that
ways are found to safeguard the confidentiality of information
given to health authorities and health professionals, while also
developing more accurate information systems for health care.

Notes

1 The Spastics Society, 62 Budge Street, Manchester M3 3BW
2 Alix Henley, Pathway Further Education Industrial Unit, Havelock Road,
   Southall, Middlesex
3 *Asian Names and Records* available from: National Extension College,
   18 Brooklands Avenue, Cambridge, CB2 2HN

4 Note the following comment: 'There is full support for any provisions which would genuinely improve communication within the NHS but the association would regret the waste of a qualified health visitor on liaison duties if these degenerated into serving only as a post box.' (Health Visitors' Association 1982)

5 Director of Nursing Services (Community), Paddington and North Kensington HA, 69 Chepstow Place, London W2

6 Network: Telephone Garston 61061

3 A better image for clinics and surgeries

'You know what going to the clinic means? Three kids to get dressed and cleaned up, 25 minutes waiting for the bus — usually in the pouring rain. And then after all that, just a row of hard benches, hours and hours of waiting and those grim yellow walls. Not a toy in sight, let alone a cup of tea. God, I dread going to the clinic.'

(Mother of three, South London)

The voice of the present echoes many from the past. For over a quarter of a century, surveys have shown that women's complaints about antenatal and child health clinics have changed little (Royal College of Obstetricians and Gynaecologists 1948; Garcia, J. 1981; Boyd, C. and Sellers, L. 1982). Then, as now, they referred to their 'cattle-market' qualities, to the length of waiting, to child care and transport difficulties and to the lack of continuity of care. Hospital antenatal clinics have been a particular focus of criticism. Clinics in general practice, though not perfect, have been commented on more favourably (O'Brien, M. and Smith, C. 1981; Cambridge Community Health Council 1977). A recent report from a working party of the Royal College of General Practioners (1982) emphasises the importance of well-designed and organised general practice premises for the parents and young children using them.

This chapter reviews a variety of ways in which all types of clinics and surgeries can be made more welcoming and attractive, especially hospital antenatal clinics. It describes schemes which show how many of the recommendations of the Maternity Services Advisory Committee 1982 for such clinics can be put into action — often with only a few cheap and simple alterations. Many of these changes come from the clinic staff themselves, who want to provide a more humane service. As a Lancashire midwife reflected: 'All mothers who attend our clinics should be made to feel very important. Somehow we have got to find the time to make them realise that even though there are dozens of other mothers and babies on our lists, they are unique . . . but perhaps we can only do that if we actually believe it ourselves.'

Reaching the clinic

'How on earth can mothers get to our clinic if they have to rely on public transport? One bus a day — if they're lucky — in most of the outlying villages. If we just left it there, we'd never see anyone.' This comment from a health visitor working in a country area was one of several which drew attention to the transport difficulties of rural families when attending clinics and surgeries (Association of County Councils 1979).

The cost of transport may also deter families from attending clinics. A senior nursing officer from Lancashire Area Health Authority wrote:

> Although patients in low income brackets may claim bus fares for attendance for essential hospital treatment, this applies only to the patient herself. Many mothers find it necessary to bring other children with them — in the case of Asians, a chaperone or interpreter will accompany the patient on almost all antenatal visits. Because these co-travellers cannot claim bus fares and because the patient is reluctant (or unable) to attend on her own, she may default.

Decentralised clinics

The Isle of Wight AHA tried to overcome these problems in their antenatal services by:

> removing some of the expense and tedium of travelling and giving expectant mothers the opportunity to see their hospital consultant obstetrician with a small team of hospital and community midwives in outlying areas. We have four such clinics and all are well attended.

The following description of antenatal clinics in Hounslow Health District shows that locally based clinics may be important in urban as well as rural areas. Such clinics have greater benefits than just being nearby. Parents often know each other and meet staff who they will see again and again. This point has been made also by GPs who run antenatal clinics for their own practices.

> For over two years we have held two decentralised antenatal clinics; one clinic is held in the centre of Hounslow, with easy access to the shops and to the buses. The other clinic is held in a part of the catchment area from which it is difficult to travel to the West Middlesex Hospital. The patients who are invited to these two clinics are the patients who find it most difficult to travel.
>
> The staff who work in the clinics are midwives from the community and from the hospital and either a Consultant or a

Senior Registrar from the hospital. They are therefore hospital clinics held in the community. We have found them very popular indeed; the patients enjoy seeing the same staff at every clinic visit, whom they get to know well. They enjoy the sense of community which is engendered in the clinic; it is their own neighbours that they meet week by week. Quite spontaneously the patients come back after the babies are born to show the staff and the other patients the new baby. Appointment systems run much more smoothly and waiting time is therefore minimal.

One criticism of this decentralised type of antenatal care is that women's medical records are more likely to get lost or be in the wrong place when they are needed (community/hospital or somewhere in between). It seems, however, that there may be a solution to this difficulty. In a study from a London teaching hospital, the women having antenatal care at a health centre where the hospital obstetricians visited were asked to look after all their own notes and records. Among these women, there were fewer notes lost or not available when needed than among a control group of women who had all their antenatal care in the hospital, and whose notes were looked after in the usual fashion by the hospital (Taylor, R.W. 1982; pers. comm.).

Mobile clinics

Mobile clinics can be another solution to families' travelling problems. Sandwell Community Health Council drew attention to their health authority's mobile immunisation unit. This is taken to areas where there is a low use of these services. A study of a similar type of mobile clinic in Southwark has shown its association with increased immunisation rates. Ormskirk District, with its large rural area, uses a mobile clinic for its community child health services. A team composed of a clinical medical officer, a health visitor and a school nurse visits the villages which are too small to justify a child health clinic and where it may be difficult to find suitable accommodation. This service is reported to be popular and well-used by people living in the country.

Transport

Several health authorities have organised transport schemes to bring parents and children into antenatal and child health clinics. Warwickshire AHA has paid for a mini-van to visit the rural areas once a fortnight with set stops to bring mothers and babies into the child health clinic. It also brings in any pregnant women in need of antenatal care.

The same health authority gives health visitors a special insurance cover for their cars so that they can drive mothers and children to clinics if they need to.

Several private transport systems were described. These have been introduced since a change in the law which now allows for payment towards the cost of journeys for lifts given in private cars which are appropriately insured. In certain mining communities in the north of England, where public transport is reported as being almost non-existent, health visitors have encouraged mothers with cars to collect and bring groups of other mothers into the clinics.

The provision of transport for those without cars is an important part of many voluntary organisations' work. Locally based voluntary groups will often help families get to clinics if they know this is needed — for instance Network, Watford (chap. 2) and Home-Start, Leicester (chap. 8). Some general practice patients' committees do this too (chap. 10).

Timing of clinics

If possible, the timing of clinic appointments should be compatible with parents' and children's life and work routines as well as those of health service staff. Though it is difficult to design clinic times to suit every member of the family, the following schemes suggest ways in which things might be improved. Although most of these examples come from hospital antenatal clinics they will often be useful in other clinic and surgery settings.

● It seems that anyone wanting to improve the timing of their clinic service should work closely with their clinic booking-clerks. Despite recommendations from the then Ministry of Health (1954), and RCOG (1982) to the contrary, some clinics still 'block book' their appointments. (In other words, they invite groups of people to come on the hour every hour throughout the clinic session.) Once the clinic has started, staff have difficulty in catching up with the backlog of patients, many of whom will have come earlier than necessary.

In trying to overcome this problem, it may be relevant to note a booking system used in an antenatal clinic in Canada (Murray Enkin, pers. comm.). It is estimated that this clinic sees an average of five patients an hour. If the clinic starts at 9.00 am, two patients are booked for 9.00 am, two for 9.15 am and one for 9.30 am. This means that the person booked for 9.00 am is seen immediately and the other four have to wait only a relatively short time before they are seen. It allows half an hour within every hour for the doctor to catch up with any backlog of patients. In this way women's waiting times are reduced.

● Some hospital antenatal clinics give the first morning appointments to mothers with young children. At this time doctors are usually up-to-date with their appointments, and toddlers may be less irritable than later in the day. This arrangement appears to work well and has the advantage that children accompanying their mothers to the clinic have other children to play with.

● Coventry Community Health Council carried out an antenatal clinic survey which suggested that mothers attending for afternoon appointments were often delayed in the clinic beyond the time when they were due to pick up their schoolchildren. Because of this, the appointment system of the local clinic has been altered to give the first appointments in the afternoon to these mothers. This type of adjustment to appointment times require that clinic booking staff are flexible, offering parents times to suit their needs.

● Several health authorities reported modifications of their routine clinic times to encourage attendance by parents who go out to work. These initiatives appear to have been in response to special local needs — for instance, in those neighbourhoods with large numbers of women working in the day or with Asian women reluctant to visit the clinic without their husbands. Sandwell and Lancashire AHAs hold evening child health clinics which are well attended. Enfield and Haringay AHA has tried an experimental clinic on the first Saturday of each month and report that it is popular and well attended.

In these three schemes, which appear to have been successful, health visitors have played a key role in advertising the service and inviting families who might find the altered clinic time convenient. I have occasionally heard, however, of evening clinics which fail to attract adequate numbers. Sometimes these failures seemed to be due to an over-estimate of the demand for such a service. They may also have been associated with poor publicity to the appropriate groups of parents.

Play for children

Many parents attending antenatal clinics and virtually all those using child health clinics bring children with them. It is surprising that facilities for children, such as toys and play areas, are still considered 'initiatives' in these services. The following examples show the range of agencies which may be involved in making clinics into better places for children.

● A mother, a member of the Pre-school Playgroups Association (PPA), recalled that with her first baby the health visitor had arranged a 'tea, chat and toys' corner in the clinic for the mothers and babies:

All went well and a noisy, untidy, happy crowd gathered regularly until the originator left and the new health visitor refused to put up with it. Despite appeals to the Senior Nursing Officer the decision was upheld and the sterile calm and peace returned to the clinic.

Another member of the PPA spoke of her antenatal clinic which, because of limited space, would not allow mothers to bring another adult or any child under five. 'What on earth do mothers do with their young children?' she asked angrily.

● In some areas voluntary organisations have started to answer this question. They have approached health service staff with offers of help to introduce play areas into the antenatal and child health clinics. These have been furnished, equipped with toys and supervised by a wide variety of agencies, such as the PPA, local branches of the Red Cross, the National Association for the Welfare of Children in Hospital, the Women's Royal Voluntary Service (WRVS), General Practices' Patients' Committees, students from local technical colleges and childminders. A few clinics have regular visits from their neighbourhood playbus. A WRVS scheme in Sussex also caters for the older children who may have to attend clinics with their parents. They provide a small library of books and hold story-telling sessions in the clinic. These volunteers feel that this type of activity encourages mothers and children to return to the clinics. (For information on the role of volunteers in antenatal clinics, see also Allen, R. and Purkis, A. 1983.)

● In many clinics it is the health service staff themselves who have been the catalysts in providing children's play facilities. Listen to this health visitor:

I think of my clinic sessions just as though I was giving a party at my own home. I'd hate to think anyone came and didn't enjoy themselves. So each week we plan a special activity — one week we have play dough, another time we borrow some water-play equipment and so on. Quite often kids come by just on the off chance that we will be having a certain activity they have taken a fancy to. It must be fun. And it must be varied so that there is always a surprise.

A senior nursing officer from Wakefield AHA went on holiday to Finland and Sweden. She was impressed by their provision of play areas in clinics. So she set about developing similar areas in all seventeen of the clinics in her district. At the start of the project the health authority contributed £100 towards buying toys and small carpet squares for the children to play on. A further £200 has been raised for toys by voluntary efforts and the sale of tea and orange juice at the clinics. In this district the play areas are not formally supervised. The informality of the children playing, often with the health visitors and parents joining in, provides ideal opportunities to discuss child development. Health visitors report that these facilities have increased the attendance rates at the child health clinics, particularly in the poorer neighbourhoods.

Several GPs describe similar schemes to provide attractive environments for the children using their surgeries. One of these, in an inner city Birmingham practice,[1] seems particularly unusual.

Attracting kids to use this surgery just isn't difficult. In fact our problem is sometimes how to get rid of them . . . For instance when one of them told me he 'couldn't possibly go to the main library 'cause that's for the rich people', I decided to set up a small children's library in the surgery waiting area. It's not very big and soon the children coming in for the books were crowding out our patients! So *that* had to be abandoned!

This GP related how he and his partner had worked with the local community group and acquired the use of a derelict site adjoining the surgery for the development of an adventure playground. Money was raised for a play leader to join the primary health care team. As the play facilities were available to all children, whether or not they attended the surgery, the play leader provided an important link between the health professionals and the local children. This increased the primary health care team's contact with the community.

These examples suggest that play facilities in clinics and surgeries can be provided with little or no cost to the health service. The main requirement is that the ideas and resources of the local community are recognised and valued. Such play facilities appear to be welcomed by parents and children. Several health care staff observed that they not only created a relaxed and friendly atmosphere which helped parents feel more at home, but they also increased the staff's job satisfaction. It should be noted, however, that several organisers of play schemes said that if the play area is too far from parents in the clinic, children may be reluctant to use it. This is particularly so if mothers are unfamiliar with the clinic and staff — a problem more likely to apply to hospital than GP clinics.

Comfort for parents

As with play for children, so with comfort for parents. How strange that simple adjustments, like soft easy chairs arranged in groups instead of lines of hard benches, and the provision of refreshments, should still be considered initiatives in services designed for parents.

Health visitors and midwives have told me how they have introduced these types of modification to their clinics. Small costs and voluntary effort by staff and local parents tend to be their hallmark.

In a few clinics, volunteer parents work with health service staff to be clinic 'welcomers' — another initiative which implies attention to the comfort of parents. Those coming to the clinic for the first time may be apprehensive, uncertain of what will be expected of them and feeling strange among so many unknown people. The job of the volunteer 'welcomer' is to identify quickly these new-comers, introduce them to the staff and other parents, tell them about the various procedures and activities in the clinic and generally try to make them feel at home. Health visitors working with such volunteers told me they thought this welcoming job is so important it should not be left to the clinic staff. They are often too busy with their clinical tasks to give it sufficient attention and time.

Continuity of care

Surveys of mothers and parents in both the antenatal and pre-school health services show that they value being able to see the same doctor, midwife or health visitor on each of their visits. Patterns of care which shuttle women and children between different clinics and teams of health professionals make it difficult for them to identify with and develop confidence in any 'key' person (Reid, M. and McIlwaine, G. 1980; Graham, H. and McKee, L. 1980).

Where antenatal clinics are decentralised, as, for instance, in some parts of Hounslow, mothers are more likely to remain with the same team of midwives, health visitors and doctors throughout their pregnancies. Consultants come out from their hospitals and visit small peripheral clinics which may be held in GPs' surgeries or health authority premises.

Continuity of care may be broken when the mother and her new baby pass from the antenatal through to the postnatal and subsequent child health services. This problem has been overcome to some extent in hospital antenatal clinics in which health visitors work alongside their midwife colleagues in seeing pregnant women. In many clinics these health visitors are the ones who care for the families when the babies are born and are back at home. A similar type of arrangement occurs in some GPs' antenatal clinics. Thus, for instance, in a Bristol general practice[2] mothers are introduced to their health visitor at their first antenatal visit and then see her on every subsequent clinic attendance during pregnancy.

An Oxford general practice[3] organises their antenatal and

postnatal clinics so that these activities all take place during the same clinic hours in the same part of the health centre. In this way parents attending during pregnancy meet other mothers who have had their babies. They are encouraged to see health care after birth as a natural continuation of antenatal care. On each occasion parents see the same health care team in familiar surroundings. The postnatal examination of the mother and the first developmental examination of the baby happen at the same clinic attendance when the baby is eight weeks old. This arrangement is more convenient for women than the usual separation of these two examinations to different clinics at different times (see also Denison, R. S. 1979).

Added attractions

Some health visitors and midwives see their clinics as places around which they can develop other activities and services for parents and young children. It could be that it is these added attractions, rather than the routine antenatal or pre-school health clinic service, which brings some parents into contact with the health clinic staff. Examples which I came across included English-language classes for Asian parents, and a drop-in centre where parents can come on any weekday, if necessary leaving their children for a few hours; also mother-and-toddler groups.

An advice centre

A health visitor from Northcote clinic, Southall wrote:

> We aim to make the clinic a focal point for anyone needing any sort of advice at any time that the clinic is open. With this in mind, we have a rota of duty officers, so that one health visitor is always on the premises and available, including lunchtime . . . an apparently simple enquiry can often lead to the discovery of a health problem.

Child health clinics may hold mother-and-toddler groups either at the same time as their clinic sessions or at other times.

Postnatal support groups

Some clinics have developed postnatal support groups . . .

> My first attempt to bring mothers (with new babies) together to make friends and share their experiences was to re-arrange the baby clinic from a queuing system to a circle of chairs where, hopefully, the mothers would sit and chat while waiting for the health visitor or doctor. However, although the mothers have conversed, the mothers I was hoping to get together did not

always come to the clinic at the same time or even the same day.

After a quick re-think, I decided to start a group on a Friday morning — despite warnings from other health visitors that similar schemes had failed. However, with the co-operation of my colleagues and nursing officers, I invited some mothers along and on a very cold October morning, seven mothers with babies of about three months arrived. Over coffee, I discussed the need for a group and they unanimously supported and re-inforced the idea. I suggested the alternatives of either a 'coffee and weather' type meeting or a more organised group with a speaker or a topic each week. They voted in favour of the latter and the group was under way.

The first week we discussed immunisation (which was a current item of concern especially regarding pertussis) and another health visitor and myself presented the facts for and against the injection. Fifteen people attended that week and despite the dreadful weather (the worst of which always seems to happen on a Friday morning), the numbers have increased and even in the worst snow, mothers have ploughed through the park with up to a maximum of thirty attending.

The mothers have themselves organised a babysitting circle and, more valuable, a list of their own names and telephone numbers for each member to keep so that if they are sitting at home during the week wishing there was somewhere to go, they can look up a nearby address and invite themselves round. This has really been a success and many firm friendships have been made. Coffee mornings and afternoons have also been organised and well attended. A newsletter is produced each month by two mothers and now when visiting new mothers I give them a copy as a welcome to the group for early involvement. Fathers often get left out in the care of their infant — so we have organised a social evening so that both parents can attend.

(Walters, M. 1979)

Ethnic minorities

Members of ethnic minority[4] communities in Britain may experience harsh inequalities of income, employment, housing and educational opportunities (House of Commons Home Affairs Committee 1981). Associated with these factors are high perinatal and infant mortality rates (Adelstein, A. *et al.* 1980). Such rates, together with the unusually young age structure of many of these communities, make them priority groups for the antenatal and pre-school child health services (OPCS 1983e).

Despite these indications of need, there are many barriers

standing in the way of these families using normal clinic services
(Homans, H. 1980).   These barriers are in addition to those
already discussed in this chapter.   For instance, the language
spoken at their clinic may be foreign and poorly understood.
Another difficulty is that the staff may know little about these
minorities' cultural customs and religious beliefs. Unintentionally,
therefore, they may offend or distress parents, particularly at
important times, such as during pregnancy and labour. A woman
Muslim community worker in Hackney wrote:

> On their first visit they have to undress completely for a general
> examination.   The Asian women beg to be seen by a woman
> doctor or midwife.   They are frightened and very nervous . . .
> they feel guilty and shameful.   They go home and ask God to
> forgive them as they never allowed themselves to be seen by a
> man other than their husband.

In some areas barriers to clinic attendance may include the fear of
racist attacks.   Health visitors in Tower Hamlets reminded me of
the Brick Lane riots in their area and more recent racist attacks on
Asian families which made them frightened to venture out in the
streets.   In other areas community health workers talked of the
anger of the black community at their unequal life chances. They
worried that a general and increasing alienation from policies and
services associated with the white majority was spilling over to
include the health services (see, for instance, Brent Community
Health Council 1981).

Health and community workers emphasise that the provision of
acceptable health services for the different ethnic communities in
this country needs great sensitivity to local racial issues on the part
of the staff, considerable flexibility in their style of working and
the ability of white health workers to listen and learn and work
with these communities and their organisations (see, for instance,
Wandsworth CRC 1978; Wandsworth and E. Merton Health
District 1979).   The following are some of the ways in which
clinics are being modified to try and make them more attractive
and acceptable.   Other schemes, such as English-as-a-second-
language courses being run concurrently with clinic sessions are
mentioned elsewhere.

Ealing, Hammersmith and Hounslow AHA has established an
antenatal clinic in an area where many Asians live.   It is staffed
with a doctor, midwife and health visitor who are all Asians, and
an English midwife who speaks Urdu.   Tower Hamlets District has
developed an informal network of contacts with doctors and
nurses returning from Voluntary Service Overseas programmes. In
this way they have attracted midwives, health visitors and clinical
medical officers with several years experience working in Sylhet

into their employment. This is the area of Bangladesh from where the majority of their Bangladeshi families come.

Interpreters

Tower Hamlets is one of several districts which has employed interpreters in their antenatal and child health clinics. Most of these are interpreters for the various Asian languages, often recruited from the local community. Some authorities are relying on volunteers or ethnic staff to do this type of work. These arrangements seem unsatisfactory both to staff and families — a point stressed in the DHSS report on Interpreter Training Needs in the NHS (Central Management Services 1982).

The views of those working with interpreters indicate that considerable skill, knowledge and sensitivity are needed by the health professionals as well as by the interpreters when working in clinics. In view of the complexity of this task, it is perhaps surprising that until recently so little attention has been given to the way in which health service interpreters can work most effectively, and the training which may be appropriate for them.

Health aides/educators

Several health authorities are employing women who speak the languages of the local ethnic minority communities to act as health aides as well as interpreters (e.g. Berkshire, Sandwell and Kirklees AHAs). One of their main qualifications for the job is that they have the trust and respect of their local communities. Usually they have no previous training as health workers. They therefore work in conjunction with health visitors and midwives who teach them about nutrition, antenatal care, child development and family planning. With this information they can act as lay health educators within their communities. They accompany and interpret for the health visitors at clinics and also during home visits. They also visit, usually on their own, new immigrant families in the area to explain about the health services and the importance of attending the clinics, and to pass on other health information which may be required. The health aides may also accompany new parents to the relevant clinics, introduce them to the health care staff and explain the reasons for the various procedures.

Health advocates

In some areas these health aides, while working in conjunction with health professionals, function relatively independently from them. They are not directly accountable to the health service and are employed and supervised by non-health service agencies. In this situation they may play the role of patient advocates —

speaking on behalf of patients and representing their interests — as well as that of lay health educators and interpreters. As advocates they asist families from the local ethnic minorities to get the type of health care which they require from the NHS. For instance, the report of the Camden Community Relations health project describes how a Bengali community worker worked in this way, advising families how to use the health services, supporting them in their contacts with clinics and introducing them to health professionals whom they need to see (Wallis, S. 1977). The knowledge which she has passed on to the local health services about this community's special health needs has been another important aspect of her advocacy work.

Multi-Ethnic Women's Health Project   A more recent development in ethnic minority health advocacy and lay health education has come from City and Hackney Community Health Council and Hackney Council for Racial Equality. The project (known as the 'Multi-Ethnic Women's Health Project'[5] has employed four women community workers with funds from the Inner City Partnership[6] and support from the health authority and Hackney Council for Racial Equality. Each woman works twenty-four hours a week. Between them they speak Turkish and four major Asian languages — Urdu, Bengali, Gujarati, Hindi and Sylheti dialect. They are supervised on a day-to-day basis by the secretary of the community health council and are supported by a steering group. This consists of roughly equal numbers of health professionals and community representatives. The workers are based at the Mothers' Hospital, Clapton, where they work in the antenatal clinics, the labour and postnatal wards. They are starting to do some group work, and are trying to visit all 'their' mothers at home at least once.

The community workers' reports on the first six months of their project suggest that there is a large demand for this service and that it is much appreciated by Turkish and Asian women:

> women coming to the clinic with emergencies and who speak no English come straight to me. It saves everybody's time and the women are seen much quicker. One such patient having a miscarriage said to me 'all my fears vanished when I saw you in the clinic as I knew that now I would be attended to without any worries'.   Zohra Ali Zubair, Health Worker

As in other projects introducing non-professionals into areas where the professions dominate (see, for instance, chap. 8), the community workers experienced initial hostility from some doctors and nurses. This came to the surface with criticisms of the need for such workers ('we've always coped adequately up till now'), their lack of 'appropriate' health care qualifications and the attendant dangers, and in issues of confidentiality. It seems, however, that these problems have quickly been overcome as the community workers have begun to help the health service staff and give them useful guidance on working with the Turkish and Asian communities. Teamwork has developed gradually as trust and work roles have become established between the professionals and non-professionals. This underlines the importance in the early stages of such projects, of giving adequate time for discussion and consultation with everyone concerned (see also chap. 9).

The steering group has become the focus for work on broader issues, including racism in the health service, eligibility and access to health care, the need for women doctors and the more sensitive deployment of medical students. One proposed initiative is the running of race-sensitivity training for hospital staff.

Health education materials for clinics

Health visitors, midwives and health education officers in areas with large ethnic minority communities have prepared a variety of health education materials for parents in the locally used languages. For instance, Hounslow Health District have made tape-slide parent craft shows, translated into the four Asian languages most commonly spoken in the district. These are meant to be shown at the antenatal clinic sessions for non-English-speaking parents. Further details of appropriate health education materials in different languages are available from the health education officers of health authorities and also from the Health Education Council, London.

A final case study

The range of initiatives described in this chapter suggest that relatively small changes to clinic organisation can improve their attraction for parents and children considerably. It seems appropriate to end with a case study which reminds one that even simple modifications of clinic routine reflect, probably more than anything else, the attitudes and work flexibility of the health care staff. The changes at the clinic show also how the energy and ideas for change in the health service often lie with the field-workers, who are closest to families' needs and wishes.

Ore clinic[7] is situated in a busy suburb containing an 'overspill' estate of families who have moved out of London. It is about two and a half miles from Hastings and adequately served by public transport and shops. The clinic, which was purpose-built some twenty years ago, is light and brightly painted and has an area which can be used for play.

The health visitors in the area are attached to primary health care teams. However, because of lack of space in their GPs' surgeries, they all work from the health authority clinic premises. Until 1979 the local child health clinic was run by one health visitor and a doctor on a weekday afternoon. Many of the health visitors felt that this was unsatisfactory as they tended to lose touch with the mothers from their own practices.

About twenty or thirty mothers came to this clinic, but the health visitors knew they were only seeing a fraction of those they needed to see. They described these sessions as 'rather formal occasions . . . the mothers sat in two lines either waiting to have their baby weighed or to see the doctor . . . the health visitor felt rushed and unable to spend her time individually with each mother.' At the suggestion of the health visitors, the nursing management agreed to change the half-day clinic into an all-day 'open-house' session. This has been running since 1979. Mothers can now come at any time, without an appointment, for help and advice or to meet friends while their children can play and be looked after. At least four health visitors, wearing their own clothes and with name badges, attend at each session. They sit and talk informally with mothers in small groups on comfortable chairs. A separate room is available for private discussion if this is needed. With the help of volunteers, coffee and tea are available for the parents and supervised play for the children.

The health visitors emphasise that one of the main objectives of this new arrangement has been to change the usual clinic relationship of the active health professional 'giving', and the passive parent and child 'receiving'. They stress the importance of listening and showing genuine interest in each child's progress. They try to involve parents actively in their child's developmental assessment, taking the time to explain the various stages of child development and the relevance of the various tests and procedures used. As it is usually too noisy for hearing tests, these are arranged on another, quieter, afternoon. Voluntary help has been found for weighing babies. This has freed the health visitors to concentrate on their health education and support role with parents.

The health visitors report that the new clinic atmosphere has been appreciated by families. Table 1 shows that the numbers of children who attended the clinic at least once in the year after the scheme began doubled when compared with the previous year. There were marked increases in every quarter. It seems likely that this improvement in attendance has been because of the changes at the clinic. The attendance figures have been collected in the same way each year and there do not appear to be any other major alterations in the population, in housing movements or in the health service to account for such large differences.

Table 1: *Numbers of children aged 0—5 years attending for the first time at Ore Child Health Clinic in 1978 and 1979*

	1978	1979
January-March	353	745
April-June	385	887
July-September	387	863
October-December	439	668
Total	1,564	3,163

The clinic health visitors commented that although these increased numbers have placed great demands on them, the change of clinic organisation has much enhanced their job satisfaction. This has probably led to a better service for families. More detailed assessments of children's development are now possible as there is less rush and plenty of time for informal observation as well as testing. Though no doctor is present at this session, health visitors refer any children they are concerned about to a separate doctors' clinic held on another day.

In conclusion

In this chapter a variety of ways have been suggested in which the 'cattle-market' image associated with many clinics — especially hospital antenatal clinics — can be countered. Small and often low-cost changes can have a surprising impact. Modification of factors such as clinic timing, play facilities for children, comfortable waiting areas for parents and attention to the language and cultural needs of ethnic minorities may improve attendance figures and also staff job satisfaction.

Attempts to change clinic practice may need to pay attention to the workload of the staff. If the nature of their task is too demanding there may be little time or energy left to experiment with new ways of working. The function of the clinic and staff roles may need to be re-examined. But whatever administrative improvements are made to enable staff to change clinic practice, the primary aim of the exercise must be kept in sight: namely to make health care more appropriate for the needs of parents and children and to do this in ways which are acceptable and attractive to them.

42   *Health for a change*

Notes

1   Dr A. Bird, The Ombersley Road Surgery, 110 Ombersley Road, Balsall Heath, Birmingham B12 8UZ
2   Dr A. Otlet, Southmead Health Centre, Wigton Crescent, Westbury-on-Trym, Bristol BS10 6PL
3   Dr K. Beswick, Didcot Health Centre, Britwell Road, Didcot, Oxfordshire OX11 7JH
4   In some areas the term 'ethnic minority' seems inappropriate. These citizens may account for a large proportion of the births — for instance nearly a quarter of all live births in Greater London (OPCS 1983a).
5   The Multi-Ethnic Women's Health Project, c/o City and Hackney CHC, 210 Kingsland Road, London E2 8EB
6   In 1977 the government established an Inner Cities Programme which related to selected inner city 'partnership' authorities (of which Hackney/Islington was one) and inner city 'programme' authorities. Extra resources have been given, through the Department of the Environment, for specified programmes to tackle urban deprivation. Health authorities have been included in drawing up these programmes.
7   Mrs Marlborough, Divisional Nursing Officer, Hasting HA, 13 Homesdale Gardens, Hastings TN34 2LY

4 Going where people are

'First take the service to where the family is. Secondly, take it in style: don't be frightened of making it pleasant and beckoning, with lots of colour and razzamatazz. Thirdly, forget your city suit, your gown and college diplomas; just join in and listen, learn and — if you can — help. And lastly remember this is the 20th century. Don't rely so heavily on the tools of yesteryear . . . Try what we have now — shops, pubs, market, holiday camps, clubs, television, local radio, telephone . . . "Only connect" as E. M. Forster reminds us on the title page of *A Passage to India*.' (Jackson, B. 1982)

Chapter 3 dealt with that part of the health service which waits for parents and children to come to them; this deals with the service reaching out. Ways are examined by which the antenatal and pre-school health services are modified to recognise the different patterns of parents' daily activities and the competing demands upon their busy lives. Health services can be introduced alongside these activities in a range of different places: in shopping centres, at childrens' daycare and at parents' work, as will be described. These are all places where the preventive health services can contact large numbers of families. Among them, there are likely to be some whom the clinic based services fail to reach.

Shopping centres

In the course of the study I have heard of several schemes which are attempting to reach people with health care in shopping centres.

● In Bolton, the community health council and health authority have initiated plans for a pregnancy walk-in clinic in the town centre to be staffed by a midwife. The position of the clinic may encourage women to obtain guidance and antenatal care earlier in their pregnancy than usual. If a woman is pregnant, the clinic will offer her immediate counselling and then refer her to her GP or hospital for regular antenatal care. Unfortunately, because of recent financial constraints, these plans have had to be postponed.

● In the 'Year of the Child' (1980) the health education department of Blackburn Health District prepared a display emphasising the importance of attending antenatal and child health clinics. Some of the large stores in the district offered to carry the display in their shop windows, free of charge. Sadly, it proved too big and was finally housed in the public library.

● Street theatre in shopping centres is another cheap way of promoting the work of the antenatal and child health services. Blackburn mentioned that they were thinking of doing this following their success working with the local comprehensive school in a health education street theatre project.

Cost is a major problem for shop-centred schemes as rates and rents in such areas are usually high and, unlike businesses, the NHS services cannot pass on the cost to their customers. When considering such programmes it may be important, therefore, to design them so they require little permanent space — for instance, mobile health clinics and health stalls in markets (Wightman, F. 1980).

Another difficulty for shop-centred health programmes is that of privacy. Schemes which offer counselling, advice or care for personal health problems should do so in surroundings which can be compatible with confidentiality. It seems that several of these programmes have been abandoned because conditions of privacy were impossible to satisfy in such places.

Pre-school nursery education and daycare facilities

As children get older their contact with child health clinics and health visitors through home visiting decreases. Yet at the ages when children are dropping out of contact with these health services, they are moving in large numbers into the orbit of pre-school nursery and daycare facilities (Dowling, S. 1978). These, then, are obvious places for the attention of the preventive child health services.

The pattern of pre-school nursery education and daycare provision varies between different parts of the country. In general, though, it is useful to distinguish between local authority services (day nurseries from social services, and nursery schools and classes from the education authorities) and the privately run services, such as playgroups and childminders. In the country as a whole only a minority of children go to the first type. For this minority, the local and health authorities usually provide examinations to check the children's health and development. The majority of children in daycare attend private services, most of these being playgroups (Osborn, A. *et al.* forthcoming). It is this type of provision which is least likely to have arrangements for regular health care and support (Dowling, S. 1980).

Establishing health service links with the many different and independent providers of daycare can be a complex and time-consuming task. The importance of such links has been emphasised in the Court and Warnock Reports and in joint circulars from the DHSS and DES calling for greater co-ordination of the pre-school child health services and all types of nursery education and day-care (DHSS and DES 1976; DHSS and DES 1978). The following are a few examples of the ways in which such integration between the child health and private daycare services is being practised.

Playgroups

Several health authorities reported close co-operation with the playgroup organisers of their social services department. A few health authorities, such as Bolton AHA and Wigan AHA, have ensured that every playgroup has a named health visitor who is responsible for visiting them and providing advice on health and childcare. The Pre-school Playgroup Association commented that such arrangements are unusual. They are concerned that many playgroups still have little or no regular contact with health visitors.

Childminders

Several authorities have made special arrangements to reach the children of working mothers who are cared for during the day by childminders. In some, such as Wigan AHA, the officer in the social services department who supervises playgroups and child-minders provides health visitors and clinical medical officers with up-to-date lists of childminders, so that they can visit them and the children in their care. The National Children's Centre in Hudders-field[1] (a voluntary organisation) runs courses for childminders and estimates they are in contact with 98 per cent of these workers in Kirklees. They also have close links with community nurses, who contribute to their courses. The staff of the centre encourage childminders to check with the parents of their children that they are seen regularly by a health visitor and at the clinic. If parents have difficulty attending clinics the childminder may obtain their permission for the child to be seen by a health visitor at the child-minder's home or at the local clinic. A 'drop-in' centre for the use of childminders in Manchester has a child health clinic, run by the health authority, once a month. Childminders appreciate this service, as it may save them attending several different clinics with the children in their care.

Playbuses

In many areas of the country, buses have been converted into playcentres where children can paint, play games, make models or whatever. The buses are bright and gaily painted and are quickly known among children in the community. The mobility of these playbuses enables them to visit neighbourhoods and estates where family support services are needed, but may not be otherwise available.

The Fundecker Playbus of the National Children's Centre in Huddersfield has a regular timetable. It is in the same place at the same time each week, providing play facilities for large numbers of children on certain council estates. Since 1978, a health visitor has joined the Playbus twice a week at lunchtime to give advice to parents and to check on the children's health and development. She works on one level of the double-decker while the children play on the other.

The workplace

Surveys have repeatedly shown that, as a group, babies from the manual social classes run higher risks of disease, disability and death than those of the non-manual social classes. Yet their parents are among those least likely to receive early and regular preventive health care either before or after their child is born (Townsend, P. and Davidson, N. 1982). By definition, the fathers of these babies are working in manual jobs, often doing unskilled work on the shop floor. Many of their mothers will also be in unskilled jobs, a large number of them being part-timers.

The workplaces of these parents are obvious targets for programmes trying to redress the social class inequalities in the availability of preventive health care and health information. In the context of health programmes for women in general, it is important to note that between 1921 and 1981 the proportion of women in the total workforce has increased from 30 per cent to 42 per cent (Rimmer, L. and Popay, J. 1982). In the last decade, when male employment levels have been falling, the proportion of women with children under five who work has remained steady. In 1980 the proportions of working women aged from sixteen to fifty-nine years with at least one child under the age of five was 23 per cent for part-timers and 7 per cent for full-timers (OPCS 1981). There are, however, large regional differences in these figures.

Loss of earnings for attending health care

At the start of this study in 1979 it seemed likely that many working women — especially those doing unskilled manual work — would be discouraged from attending antenatal and child health clinics because of loss of pay, difficulty in taking regular time off during shift work and the fear of dismissal, or transfer to less remunerative work. At that time working women and men had no legal rights for paid time off from work for any type of health care.

Now, as I finish the study in 1982, all working women have the right to reasonable paid time off work for antenatal care (the Employment Act 1980).[2]

At one level one might say that this change in the law came about because of the concern among ministers and members of the House of Commons Social Services' Committee (1982) to find ways of reducing the country's perinatal mortality rate. Yet their willingness to consider the importance of working parents' health care seems also to reflect the evidence and publicity which arose from the research and campaigns of the trade union movement and the Spastics Society. Their findings and views on the need to change the Employment Act were presented to the House of Commons Social Services' Committee when they were preparing their report on perinatal mortality (1982). This story of influence and change in the law is so important — and, at the time, seemed so unlikely — it should be recalled.

The TUC's promotion of workplace health education

For many years women in the trade union movement have attempted to promote the health of women workers through collective action at the workplace. Campaigns have included those for free and easily available contraception and for screening for cervical cancer (TUC 1981). In 1979 the Trade Union Congress became actively involved in the promotion of antenatal care and health education through the workplace. They approached the Health Education Council (HEC) for assistance with health education materials in any local workplace project which a union might initiate. This the HEC agreed to do, through health education officers. Later that year the TUC's Women's Advisory Committee prepared a paper on perinatal mortality. This stressed the importance of improving women's knowledge about health in pregnancy and suggested that local unions should negotiate with their management and health authority to set up workplace health education projects for women workers. The committee were careful not to suggest any standard ways in which this could be done. They described instead a variety of different approaches which might suit or be modified for particular work situations. The general secretary of the TUC sent this paper to twelve unions, with large women memberships in manual grades, in areas of the country with high perinatal mortality rates. He urged them to consider what action they could take locally.

The Spastics Society's promotion of workplace health education

During the time of these TUC developments the Spastics Society were running their 'Save a Baby' campaign. They were exploring the possibilities of using the workplace as a way of reaching women with health education and care in pregnancy, particularly those regarded as being 'at risk' of perinatal and infant mortality (House of Commons Social Services Committee Vol. IV. 1980).

Two major workplace antenatal care projects resulted from this initiative — one in Strathleven, Scotland and one in Oldham, England. Although this study is limited to England and Wales, the Scottish scheme is outlined because of its influence on the development of workplace health education projects in England and Wales.

Strathleven Bonded Warehouses Ltd   In mid-1979 the Spastics Society approached Strathleven Bonded Warehouses Ltd[3] to ask if they would establish a scheme to help reduce the high rates of perinatal mortality in their area.   Strathleven Bonded Warehouses employ a large female workforce of some 800 women who are mainly occupied in the unskilled manual work of bottling, blending and distributing whisky.   The Spastics Society briefed Strathleven's management on the importance of antenatal care, good nutrition and the reduction of stress in pregnancy.   They were quick to see how they could contribute to better health in these areas.   With the company's approval, an officer of the society visited their two main plants to investigate the problems of pregnant workers and to hear the views of employees, supervisors, nurses, shop stewards and management.   The officer also discussed the proposed project with representatives of the Health and Safety Executive.

Within a few months negotiations between the company's management, the General and Municipal Worker's Union, the Argyll and Clyde Health Board and the Spastics Society were completed and the workplace scheme started.   *All* female employees were informed of the scheme and told of the importance of care before birth, and to give special attention to nutrition and protection against German measles.   This was done by means of a letter which was enclosed in every female employee's paypacket.   Articles describing the scheme were published in the company newspaper, *Inbond*.

The Strathleven project now offers pregnant women health education and counselling sessions during working hours and gives a variety of incentives for them to report their pregnancy to the company's medical staff.   These incentives include paid time off to attend antenatal clinics (at the start of the project this was not a statutory right), free milk or orange juice daily, earlier finishing times to avoid the stress of the rush hour, use of a rest room at work, and alternative lighter duties, during pregnancy, if needed.

It is estimated that the scheme costs less than £1,500 for the twenty-four or so pregnancies in the company each year.   This covers the cost of free milk and the time given over to health education and attendance at clinics. The director of the company's personnel department emphasises, however, that the scheme has also brought considerable benefits and savings in improved labour relations and by reductions in the time lost through ill-health.

Perhaps because of its popularity with management, workers and the health authority, this workplace scheme continues to develop, expand and extend its influence. Now, for instance, fathers who are also employees of the company can be involved in certain parts of the scheme. When necessary they may attend clinics with their partners without loss of pay. After the birth the 'Strathleven babies' and their parents receive congratulation cards and flowers from the company.

As a direct result of this antenatal scheme, several other health education workplace projects have started in the company with the workers, management and the health care staff all working together. These include a project for problem drinking and alcoholism, and another to develop policies to prevent and ameliorate problems of disablement at work. For their part, the health board have created an additional health education officer's post for someone to work with industry and commerce, setting up further workplace health promotion schemes.

Park Cakes Ltd, Oldham   Following the success of the Strathleven scheme, the Health Education Officer in Oldham Area Health Authority,[4] together with the Spastics Society, initiated a similar project with a local manufacturer of cakes. Oldham had a high perinatal mortality rate compared with many other parts of the country. The workforce of Park Cakes, Ltd, comprises some 1,700 persons, of whom some 80 per cent are women, mainly occupied in unskilled work. Approximately 60 per cent of the workforce are of childbearing age.

Negotiations between the company's management, the Bakers and Allied Foods Union, the Spastics Society and Oldham AHA began in the autumn of 1979. As in Strathleven, management were concerned to help once they understood the nature of the problems. They had not known about the increased risk of perinatal death for the babies of manual working-class women in their area. Nor, perhaps, had they fully appreciated the difficulties of their workers who, at that time, lost money for attending antenatal clinics.

With remarkable speed the project was set up, starting in January 1980. Through the company's newly formed occupational health department, it provides (in paid time) a programme of health education and counselling to all pregnant employees for an hour every week on Friday afternoons. Part-time and full-time women workers are encouraged to attend till they leave to have their babies. There are talks, discussions and films on many aspects of pregnancy and the development of the baby, often with outside speakers, such as local health visitors and midwives. Since the start of the project this counselling and advice service has been extended to make it available to workers on an informal 'drop-in' basis during any of their work breaks. Ex-employees sometimes return to the occupational health department for advice. Occasionally male employees, new to fatherhood, seek advice for wives who are not employed by the company.

The company also gives pregnant women paid leave for antenatal clinic visits (now a statutory right), rubella screening, subsidised canteen meals and the right to leave work early to avoid rush-hour travel. Lighter duties can be arranged for those working at the bakery, particularly for those working near the hot ovens where the heat and sweet smell of the bread may be a problem.

Although the scheme is voluntary, in its first two years most of the known pregnant employees have made use of the paid time off to attend antenatal clinics. Attendance at the Friday afternoon counselling and health education sessions has been almost 100 per cent. The main exceptions are part-timers who are not in the factory on that afternoon.

Seventy-seven pregnant women enrolled in the scheme between January 1980 and January 1982. A 'snapshot' profile of the social characteristics of the women taking part at one point in time (mid-1980) showed that out of the thirteen, three were single mothers, five were teenagers and ten were considered to be in social classes 4 and 5 (as measured by their husband's occupation), with the majority being in the latter social class. Several of the women were Bengali-speaking Asians. This social profile of the women using the workplace scheme appears to have remained fairly typical.

In obstetric terms all of these women are in 'high risks' groups, often having difficult social circumstances and with an increased risk of perinatal mortality. Park Cakes, through their counselling and health education services, is providing them with more support and information than is offered to most other pregnant women. This is a good example of positive discrimination of health care in favour of those most likely to need it.

Some problems   Those initiating these two schemes have reported only one major problem, namely that of allaying the anxiety of GPs and obstetricians that they are setting up a rival service. They have had to emphasise repeatedly that they are only trying to increase the women's awareness of the role and importance of NHS antenatal care and their own knowledge of health in pregnancy.

With time, it seems that many of these doctors have grown to trust the scheme as they have been involved in the companies' counselling and health education sessions and have come to know the occupational health staff through their referrals. However, one of the companies reported that in their area the GPs are still conspicuous for their lack of support and are sometimes even in frank opposition to the scheme. This antagonism may be due partly to their fear of losing income — GPs are paid a fee for each patient they provide with antenatal care. It is also aggravated by the company's refusal to pay them a fee for any involvement in the health education sessions. This is just one of several examples I have encountered during this study that suggests that the way in which GPs are paid may make it difficult for them to work flexibly with other agencies in preventive health care. Health visitors, midwives, health education officers and community physicians, all of whom receive a salary which is unaffected by the type of work they do or the number of patients they deal with, are now enthusiastic supporters of this scheme.

But perhaps a more fundamental problem of these models for workplace health promotion has been raised by the TUC (House of Commons Social Services Committee Vol. IV 1980). They point out that the crucial people in the Strathleven and Oldham projects are the occupational nursing staff. A study carried out in 1976 by the Employment Medical Advisory Service indicated that a large proportion of firms (85 per cent of their sample) employ no occupational health staff at all (Health and Safety Commission, 1978). To quote the TUC:

> We do not believe it is the job of employers as a general rule to employ skilled staff to provide basic medical services which duplicate that provided by the NHS . . . The TUC would wish to emphasise, therefore, that they would hope that future health education projects would be more closely linked into the preventive and curative services provided locally by the NHS. This might mean that projects were located in clinics or health centres rather than the workplace itself. This might, in any event, be a more appropriate solution for a joint project involving a number of small employers in an industrial estate within a closely circumscribed industrial area. More probably, it would mean health authority staff — particularly health visitors, midwives, community physicians, dieticians and health education officers, going into workplaces and holding sessions in suitable rooms within the workplace. Assuming full support from the employer, this would ensure high takeup of high quality services.
>
> (TUC Memorandum to House of Commons Social Services Committee on Perinatal and Neonatal Mortality. 1980)

Disseminating information about workplace health projects

Publicity and the dissemination of information about workplace antenatal projects has been an important feature of the work of the Spastics Society, a few employers (notably Strathleven Bonded Warehouses Ltd) the TUC and the Health Education Council. The Spastics Society have worked extensively with the press, radio and television to publicise the findings and experience of their various workplace antenatal schemes.   The Strathleven Company has produced an information pack[5] for others interested in starting similar schemes.   Working with the Scottish Health Education Group, they have also produced a video film about ways of promoting workplace health education schemes.[6]   For their part, the TUC have used their various information networks to contact workers around the country, telling them what these schemes can offer and the different ways in which they can be set up.

Recent developments in workplace health projects

As a result of all this publicity, these organisations have received many enquiries from companies and unions throughout the country interested in setting up their own workplace schemes. It appears however, that few other workplace projects have been established on the scale of the Strathleven or Park Cakes schemes.

Since 1980, the main development in workplace health schemes for pregnancy and early childhood seems to have been an increase in negotiated arrangments between management and unions to establish more than the new statutory minimum for women's health rights in pregnancy.   The range of these agreements is wide and includes all the different features of the Strathleven and Park Cakes schemes (for instance early leaving, lighter duties and nutrition supplements).   A few companies also provide free transport to antenatal clinics or reimburse the travelling costs; others offer all their female employees free rubella testing and vaccination (TUC 1982).

It is important to note, however, that these agreements rarely take into account the needs of parents to attend to the health of their children, once born. This is an omission which needs correcting. A survey of pregnant women in West London showed that a high proportion of them intended to return to paid employment after the birth (Rodmell, S. and Smart, L. 1982).   Children's vulnerability to premature death, disease and disability is not confined to their first nine months of existence *in utero*. Just taking deaths, some 70 per cent of all deaths between birth and the age of fifteen occur in the first year of life (OPCS 1980). As in pregnancy there seems great scope for workplace-centred health education, advice and counselling services concerned with supporting parents in the health care of their children. Employers could also enable working parents to attend necessary clinics and surgeries for their children's health and developmental surveillance and immunisation and also for their care when they are ill. And here, as in the pregnancy schemes, it is important to include fathers as well as mothers, for they too have rights and duties in matters of their children's health.

And thinking of the future, it is worth drawing attention to an observation of the Maternity Alliance and Islington Community Health Council (1981). They point out that the NHS is itself in a good position to set an example to other industries as a progressive employer of pregnant women. It is the largest employer in the country and the majority of its workers are women. Yet it appears to have a poor reputation for looking after the health of its workers. A survey of some 6,000 pregnant women throughout the country commented on the difficulties at work for NHS employees (Boyd, C. and Sellers, L. 1982). Complaints were frequently made by nurses. During their pregnancies they had to continue with their usual stressful workload, undertaking heavy physical tasks such as lifting, and being exposed to infections. If health authorities could stand out as employers who take great care of their own workers' health, this might encourage other employers to emulate health promoting schemes in their workplaces.

In conclusion

A greater proportion of the population may be reached with health care in pregnancy and early childhood if the services are taken to places frequented by large numbers of parents and their children: particularly those who do not tend to use preventive services. Attention could be given to the place of employment of women workers, especially those in manual occupations; also to the main providers of daycare for young children, particularly the children of lone and employed parents who may have difficulty attending daytime clinics. The chances of developing these types of 'opportunistic' approaches to reach families with potential health problems will vary from place to place and might include the large annual gatherings of gypsies at their horsefairs (chap. 8) and units for homeless families (chap. 2).

Notes

1 The National Children's Centre, Longroyd Bridge, Huddersfield, West Yorkshire
2 For a useful checklist of maternity rights see 'Pregnant at Work — a

Checklist for Employers, Personnel Officers and Trade Union Representatives', available from Maternity Alliance, 309 Kentish Town Road, London NW5 2TJ. See also 'Maternity Rights for Working Women' by Jean Coussins, available from NCCL, 21 Tabard Street, London SE1

3   Alistair Robertson, Director and Head of Personnel, Strathleven Bonded Warehouses Ltd, Gooseholm, Dumbarton G82 2SB

4   Health Education Officer (Commerce and Industry), Oldham HA, St Peter's House, Oldham OL1 1JT

5   Available from Personnel Dept. Strathleven Bonded Warehouses Ltd. (See note 3.)

6   'The Fight Against Perinatal Death and Handicap — What Industry Can Do' can be borrowed free of charge from the Scottish Health Education Group, Woodburn House, Canaan Lane, Edinburgh EH10 4SG.

5 Out-of-hours preventive services from midwives and health visitors

'OK when there's obviously something wrong. But what about that small bleed I had in the seventh month? . . . would the baby still be all right in the morning? I hardly slept that night. And when Jo burnt his hand — that was an emergency. But that night he screamed and screamed and nothing I could do would settle him. God, I needed help. He was going mad and so was I. I had visions of something awful going on in his stomach . . . surgeons having to operate . . . Then I thought, don't be hysterical. They'll only say it's his teeth. All babies scream. But how does one know when it's serious? There's so much about cot deaths now. Things happen so quickly when they're babies . . . I'd just love someone I could whisper my worries to without really disturbing them. Just some signal to know that I was doing the right thing. But I'd be frightened to bother a doctor — what would he say if it was nothing?' (A first-time mother, London)

The last chapter concerned the extension of the range of places where preventive health services are offered to families in pregnancy and early childhood. This chapter discusses ways of extending the range of times when these services are available. The need for such extensions has been emphasised in a variety of important reports concerning family health: the Court Report (1976), the Report of the Select Committee on Violence in the Family (1977) and the Children's Committee Report on Out-of-Hours Social and Health Care (1980).

Anyone who has worked as a GP or in a casualty department will be only too aware of the round-the-clock cover which exists for all types of problems in pregnancy and early childhood. But talk to parents and you will get a different story. 'Out-of-hours' are the times when surgeries and offices are usually closed: evenings, nights, weekends and bank holidays. These are often the only times when parents who work and children who are out at daycare during the week can receive their routine home visits from midwives and health visitors. They may also be the only times when such families can attend clinics and health education sessions. And if parents have a sudden and unexpected problem with their pregnancy or child during these 'out-of-hours' times it may be difficult to find an appropriate source of advice and help, other than the emergency GP and casualty services.

I will now describe ways in which some midwives and health visitors are trying to modify the way in which they work to provide out-of-hours services of a mainly preventive nature. Inevitably these services will occasionally detect acute medical emergencies needing curative treatment, perhaps even hospital care. Even here, though, they may perform a preventive function (known as 'secondary prevention'), picking up illness early and enabling medical intervention to occur as soon as possible. This may affect and improve the course and outcome of the disease. In a few cases it may even save lives.

Extended preventive midwifery services

The hospital midwifery services provide a 24-hour, 7-day-a-week service for births and for women needing in-patient antenatal and postnatal care. In contrast, the availability of routine advice, health education and surveillance for pregnant women outside hospitals and outside normal clinic hours is sometimes less extensive.

It seems, though, that the 'out-of-hours' community midwifery services which health authorities plan and pay for are often different from those which midwives carry out unofficially and voluntarily in their own time. Many midwives told me that they visit women who work during the day, at evenings and weekends. Some give mothers their home 'phone numbers so they can be contacted if they are worried or if there is an emergency. This extra work is frequently carried out in addition to midwives' normal workload, with no financial reward.

Nottingham's extended midwifery services

Several districts, however, described how their community midwifery services are planned and organised to encourage and remunerate community midwives for making their services as accessible as possible to women at all times in their pregnancies. In North Nottingham District, for instance, this is achieved mainly through a series of home visits. A minimum of three is recommended. Whenever possible the midwives make appointments with the mothers so that the visits fall at times which are convenient for them. If parents are only at home in the evenings or at weekends the midwives are paid extra for visiting them at these times.

At the first visit the mother is given a daytime 'phone number where she can phone and leave messages for her own midwife to call her back. She is also given an emergency number through which she can contact an 'on-call' midwife at any time, including nights, Saturdays, Sundays and bank holidays. This 'phone is manned by staff of Ambulance Control, who can contact the duty midwives by means of their 'pocketfone' radios. All midwives are expected to do a period of time covering this 'on-call' service.

'Dial-a-midwife' services in Shropshire and West Berkshire

Shropshire[1] and West Berkshire District[2] have another type of 'dial-a-midwife' community service, based on GP maternity units. Though both these schemes have developed independently of each other, they appear remarkably similar in their orientation and organisation. I will therefore describe only one of them in detail, namely the West Berkshire scheme (see also Page, N. E. 1978; Waterhouse, I. 1977).

After the reorganisation of the NHS in 1974, the community midwifery services in West Berkshire District were integrated with those of the old hospital midwifery division. This resulted in the management of the local midwifery services being based on each of the four GP maternity units, each of which is situated in a different sector of the district. This new integrated midwifery service combines the resources of the domiciliary service with those of the GP unit. It is under the management of one nursing officer and serves all the population in the geographical sector around the unit. Among other things it provides a 24-hour advisory and support service for parents, which can be contacted through the GP unit's switchboard.

Parents are told of the dial-a-midwife service when midwives make their first home visit. They are given a card on which is clearly printed the 'phone number of the midwife attached to the woman's general practice and the emergency number of their local GP unit. Parents are told that they can 'phone at any time of day or night, no matter how trivial they think their problem is. Midwives in the GP unit are up and working through the night. 'Phone calls at this time — or any other — will not disturb them.

The nursing officer who established the service emphasised the importance of adequate time for coping with parents' anxieties. She recalled her own experience when working on a busy consultant unit labour ward. When parents called for advice the midwives were usually too rushed with their ward work to give them the necessary attention. The workloads of the midwives on the GP labour wards are much less than these consultant units and allow midwives to counsel and advise worried parents without being rushed. If necessary a midwife visits the family immediately.

In both Shropshire and West Berkshire, the midwives' records suggest that there has been a considerable increase in the number of calls since the start of the services in 1975. By 1980 the West Berkshire scheme was receiving an average of 152 calls a month.

About a third of the callers were visited by a midwife at home. Mothers are the main users of the service, though it is not unusual for fathers to 'phone in. The majority of the calls are from parents after the birth of their baby, although the number of calls received from pregnant mothers appears to be increasing. When there was press publicity about the possible dangers of the drug Debendox in pregnancy, the Shropshire project reported a marked increase in 'phone calls from pregnant mothers. These were often very late at night, with mothers wanting to know whether they had been prescribed this drug and its possible effects on their baby.

In Shropshire this dial-a-midwife service only extends until the baby's twenty-eighth day. After this, parents are referred to their health visitor or some other appropriate source of help. In West Berkshire, however, calls and visits are made to children of any age, although they are rarely older than one year. The relevant information is passed on to the health visiting service the next day. This unusual extension of the midwifery support service into the normally accepted professional territory of health visitors has occurred with the full agreement of the local health visitors and midwives. With this extended midwifery service, closely co-ordinated with the health visitors, there is apparently no need for an out-of-hours health visiting service.

Extended health visiting services

Health visiting has traditionally been organised to cover only the daytime working hours, Monday to Friday. As with midwives, though, it seems that many health visitors voluntarily extend their work beyond these times, visiting parents in the evenings and giving them their home 'phone numbers for use in times of crisis. This may be particularly important in rural areas where families often live many miles from their nearest health centre or hospital. A few predominantly rural health authorities, such as Devon AHA, encourage this extension of the health visitors' work by paying the cost of their telephone installation and rental.

In recent years several urban districts have organised their health visiting services to extend to evenings, nights, weekends and bank holidays. I identified seven of these schemes, the first of which was set up in Huddersfield District[3] in 1977 (see table 2). A few, such as those of Enfield[4] and Huddersfield District seem securely established. Others such as Colchester[5], Harrow[6] and Plymouth District[7] have been short-lived experiments which ceased for lack of adequate funding and staffing.

Table 2 shows the variation in the way these different schemes have been organised. All of them have shared common objectives: the reduction of morbidity and mortality in early childhood from

Table 2: *Some out-of-hours health visiting services**

Name of project	Length of operation	Cover of phone-in advisory service Hours		Other key characteristics
		Weekdays	Weekend and bank holidays	
Barnet/Finchley Week-End Extended Health Visiting Service	March 1979—	Nil	Extended day-time service. Each day: (9.00—20.00)	Staffed by day-time volunteer HVs. Also includes routine home visiting.
Colchester Extended Health Visiting Service	1977 for 1 year	Nil	24 hours bank holidays and weekends only.	Staffed by day-time volunteer HVs.
Enfield Extended Health Visiting Service	March 1979—	Evenings/nights (19.00—8.30)	24 hours each day	Staffed by additional paid staff. Also includes routine home visiting, evening clinic and health education services.
Harrow Pilot 24-hour Health Visiting Service	June 1978— March 1979	Evenings/nights (18.00—7.00)	Evenings each day (18.00—23.00)	Staffed by day-time volunteer HVs.
Huddersfield Crying Baby Advisory/Relief Service	April 1977—	Evenings/nights (19.00—7.00)	24 hours each day	Staffed by day-time volunteer HVs.
Kingston and Richmond Crying Baby Scheme	Oct 1979— 1981	Nil	24 hours each day	Staffed by day-time volunteer HVs. No home visiting allowed.
Plymouth Pilot Crying Baby Service	June 1979— Nov 1979	Evenings (18.00—23.00)	Evenings each day (18.00—23.00)	Staffed by day-time volunteer HVs.

*Information compiled mid-1980

all causes, but especially from non-accidental injury and sudden infant death. To quote from the evaluation report of the Huddersfield Crying Baby Advisory/Relief Service:

we were hopeful that the scheme, technically at least, would be capable of rendering preventable those cases of non-accidental injury to children which occur when a number of stressful factors exist within the family and a persistently crying child acts as a flashpoint. It could also provide some relief for anxious parents, in that the knowledge that assistance of this kind is immediately available may well have a positive effect on the emotional stability of the family. In addition, help of this kind could perhaps prevent relatively insignificant issues assuming enormous proportions.   (Kirklees AHA 1977)

The information on which I am drawing derives from health visitor records which several of the schemes have used to monitor the number and nature of the calls received. In addition, Huddersfield, Plymouth and Harrow carried out surveys of parents using their services at the start of their schemes (Kirklees AHA 1977; Bogie, A. 1981; Parrick, M. 1979). People who called the service were asked to complete questionnaires giving details such as the composition of their families, their situation when they called the service, the outcome of their calls and their satisfaction with the service.

The numbers of families involved in each of these surveys were fifty-six in Huddersfield, seventy-one in Plymouth, and eighty-four in Harrow. These figures represent response rates of 70 per cent, 86 per cent and 68 per cent respectively. The research was carried out by health visitors in the course of their everyday work and also in their free time.

What was offered

During the times that they were open, all seven of these extended health visitor schemes have provided a 'phone-in service which parents can use to contact a health visitor if they have been anxious about their child, or needed advice. Kingston and Richmond AHAs[8] have been the only schemes where counselling, advice and referral to other agencies have been carried out entirely by telephone. This restriction was introduced to protect health visitors' safety. Elsewhere health visitors have been allowed to respond to the calls with home visits. In most of the schemes about half the calls resulted in a home visit.

In addition to these 'phone-in advisory services, the Enfield and the Barnet/Finchley[9] Extended Health Visiting Services have provided out-of-hours routine home visiting for families who cannot be contacted during weekdays. The Enfield scheme, which has been the only one to employ additional staff for its out-of-hours services, has also provided evening clinics and health education sessions (Haylock, M. 1981; Harrington, C. 1981).

Advertising

Most of the projects described their method of advertising as 'low-key'. Midwives and health visitors have told parents about the service during their antenatal and postnatal visits. They have usually given them a card describing the times covered by the service and the 'phone number to contact. Posters with similar information have been displayed in clinics and surgeries. None of the schemes has used the local press or radio for regular advertising. In places where the service has been established for some years, such as Huddersfield, health visitors report that many local parents know of its existence through hearing other parents talk about it.

How the services worked

The 'phone number given for most of these out-of-hours advisory services has been that of the local hospital or ambulance station. Such switchboards have the advantage of being open day and night, every day of the year. On receiving a parent's call, the switchboard contacts the duty health visitor at home by 'phone or by GPO bleep. The health visitor then contacts the parents. By this method health visitors have kept their home 'phone numbers private. The duty health visitors record details of all calls received. On the next working day, they inform the family's own health visitor about the presenting problems and any action that they have taken.

The Enfield scheme has differed from this pattern. At 7.00 p.m. from Monday to Friday, the duty health visitor reports to her base, which is situated in the antenatal department at the District General Hospital. Here she collects details of any home visits referred by the daytime staff. Urgent 'phone calls from parents reach her here or, while out visiting, by means of the hospital switchboard and her 'bleep'. When the evening visits are over the duty health visitor returns to the hospital and sees parents and children on the maternity and paediatric wards. At 11.00 p.m. she returns home where she is on call via her 'bleep' till 8.30 a.m. During the week a second health visitor is on call from home to take parents' 'phone calls when the other health visitor is busy. During weekends and bank holidays only one health visitor is on call from home by 'bleep'.

Nature of calls received

The number of calls received by a 'phone-in advisory service reflects many factors, such as the size of the population covered, the way the service is advertised, its staffing and the number of hours it is available. Unfortunately, none of the data available from the schemes has been analysed to take account of these factors. However, it is interesting to note that in the first months of the Huddersfield and Plymouth schemes the number of calls they received were very similar — an average of about three a week. Within two years the number of calls received by the Huddersfield service trebled, suggesting that with time people hear about the service and learn to use it. Both these schemes have been run by volunteer health visitors in their spare time. The Enfield scheme received many more referrals than this, amounting to some 1,200 in the first year. This may have been because of its special staffing and the other extended home visiting services provided.

In both the Plymouth and Colchester schemes health visitors designed their services bearing in mind the many armed forces' families in their districts. From their routine health visiting they knew that many of these young mothers were under considerable stress with their husbands away on dangerous tours of duty. In addition, they were often very isolated, being a long way from their own families and friends. It is not surprising, therefore, that the evaluation of the first six months of the Plymouth Crying Baby Scheme showed that over a third of the callers were service families. The majority of them were naval. Most of the mothers were under twenty-one years of age. All of them were at home on their own at the time of their calls.

Several potential criticisms of these types of 'out-of-hours' 'phone-in services should be considered. First there is the possibility that they might be swamped through excessive use by mothers working during the day. This was not borne out by the Huddersfield evaluation of its first six months of operation. Only four of the eighty mothers who called the service in this time were working in a full- or part-time capacity. This figure was considerably less than expected from the known rate of mothers with pre-school children who work.

Next there is the criticism that the people who are most in need of help are the least likely to have their own telephone or be sufficiently confident, when anxious, to use a 'phone to contact the service. Though this may often be true, it should be noted that 19 per cent of the Huddersfield calls came from 'phone boxes. A further 12 per cent were from 'phones outside the families' homes, such as those of their neighbours. In Plymouth as many as 40 per cent of the calls came from 'phone boxes.

It is also sometimes said that parents who are reluctant to use the routine antenatal and child health services are unlikely to use this type of out-of-hours service. Once again, this may be true in many instances. But in the first six months of the Huddersfield scheme at least three of the eighty mothers who 'phoned had not received any antenatal care at all.

The projects reported that most of their calls concerned babies of less than six months. Parents were often extremely anxious; the majority 'phoned because they could not stop their baby crying. The exact nature of the underlying problem in the child was sometimes difficult to define accurately over the telephone. The reports of the Harrow, Huddersfield and Plymouth projects suggest, however, that the commonest cause was feeding problems. These were sometimes from mothers who were breast-feeding. Sometimes they were due to inappropriate bottle feeding — perhaps too much or too little. Occasionally the babies had colds that caused difficulty in sucking. On a couple of occasions help was needed to feed a baby with a cleft palate. Going through the records of some of these services, many other types of worries were revealed which, if left through the long hours of the night and weekend, might have resulted in extreme anxiety. A few could have been early warning signals of more serious problems:

Mother in tears because cut finger of baby while cutting her nails. Visited. Very small superficial graze on left side of index finger by the nail. No other sign of injury. First time parents in need of reassurance and support.

Blood in baby's stool. Referred to GP.

Premature baby discharged home on New Year's Eve after a mid-thigh amputation of right leg. Parents very anxious and lacking in confidence. Visited twice on New Year's Day to give support and advice.   (Extracts from records of the
Barnet/Finchley Extended Health Visiting Service)

Parents' response

The general impression of health visitors has been that parents welcome these out-of-hours visiting and advice services but have been surprised that they exist. The fear that they might be misused does not appear to have been borne out by the experience of any of the projects examined. Health visitors felt that virtually all their calls have been ones which should be dealt with by their profession. Parents using the Plymouth scheme were asked who they would have contacted if the service had not existed. About half the families said that they would have contacted their GP. However, none of the health visitors spoken to in this or other schemes felt that they were providing an alternative service to that of the GPs. The opening of two of the projects coincided with the withdrawal of the local social work out-of-hours emergency service. Health visitors emphasised that they did not receive any calls about what they felt were purely social work problems.

Staffing and remuneration

With the exception of the Enfield project, these extended health visiting services have not employed extra staff. They have relied on 'volunteers' from their normal daytime establishment to cover the unsocial hours of the service. In Barnet/Finchley District about 50 per cent of the health visiting staff have worked in the project. In Huddersfield the proportion has been about 30 per cent and in the Plymouth pilot project only 25 per cent were involved, although 50 per cent volunteered. Work rotas have been organised so that the 'volunteers' are on call as infrequently as possible.

In Enfield a separate staff of health visitors have been employed for the night or weekend work. To quote the nursing manager who initiated the scheme:

From my own experience I knew the strain of carrying a large caseload which had fluctuated over the years from 900 to 450 families. After a day of coping with that kind of caseload, evening visits were not looked upon with pleasurable antici-
pation.   (Haylock, M. 1981)

By 1980 Enfield were employing five part-time health visitors to cover their 'out-of-hours' services. They were all mothers with young children who welcomed the opportunity of maintaining their professional expertise while their children were growing up.

The extent of the health visitors' remuneration in the 'voluntary' schemes varied. Most have been paid in accordance with the Whitley Council agreement for being on call during unsocial hours (Nurses and Midwives Council 1976, pt IV, para 229). This amounts to £1.50 for 8.00 p.m. to 8.00 a.m.; £2.25 for the whole of Saturday and Sunday; and £3.00 for public holidays. If health visitors make home visits they are sometimes given time off in lieu or are paid only their normal hourly rate. They all have their travelling expenses paid. Some health authorities have paid for the cost of telephone installation and rental as well as the 'phone calls which health visitors make in the course of their work. In addition, Enfield, Barnet/Finchley and Kingston and Richmond Districts have given their health visitors GPO bleeps, thus saving them the restriction of staying in their homes when they are on call.

Costs

In 1979 the Huddersfield project, which covered every night, weekend and bank holiday was estimated to cost 61 per cent of one health visitor's salary (midpoint) a year. The cost of the six months of the Plymouth pilot scheme, also in 1979, amounted to approximately £700. Both these schemes have been run by volunteer health visitors: no extra staff have been employed. The cost of the Enfield scheme for the year between March 1979 and February 1980 was approximately £6,500. This covered the salaries of five part-time health visitors, their car allowance, telephone expenses (including rental) and the cost of the GPO radio paging service.

Some problems

Though many health visitors feel these extended services are needed, there are several problems which may inhibit their further development. For instance, several inner city authorities are concerned about the safety of health visitors going out to visit families at night. This is the reason why the Kingston/Richmond service was restricted to over-the-phone counselling, advice and referrals. In another of the schemes the health visitors have been issued with assault alarms. In yet another, the ambulance control switchboard call the health visitors at frequent intervals to check that they are safe when out visiting.

The most serious problems, however, appear to be those associated with the health visitors' conditions of work in the schemes relying on 'volunteer' staff. Their fees and reimbursement of expenses are so small that they are neither a financial incentive nor a compensation for the inconvenience of having to work unsocial hours. There have also been reports of exhaustion from overwork. In all but the Enfield scheme, health visitors have carried out these duties in addition to their full daytime work schedules. Nursing managers report that the demand for their normal daytime service is often so great that they can give health visitors time off in lieu for the extra work only if the service is given extra staff. In such situations they are concerned that these 'out-of-hours' schemes may threaten the efficiency of their normal daytime health visiting services.

The report of the Harrow scheme (Parrick, M. 1979) gave both these difficulties as reasons why their scheme, if it continued, should employ separate 'out-of-hours' staff. In its limited nine months of operation, the number of volunteer health visitors decreased from twenty to eight. To quote a nursing officer: 'You can run a service on goodwill for so long, but after a while you stretch it too far.' The Harrow scheme also revealed the inconvenience of these schemes to health visitors' own families if they are not provided with 'bleeps'. Health visitors had to stay near telephones during the evenings and weekends. 'Often husbands were left consoling crying children disturbed by the telephone, whilst their mother was out dealing with the crying baby of another family.'

The Enfield scheme, which pays additional out-of-hours staff to run the service, has not experienced any of these problems concerned with health visitors' working conditions. It seems an important model for future developments in this type of service.

In conclusion

The experience of this study suggests that many midwives and health visitors feel there is a need for 'out-of-hours' preventive health services which can be contacted easily by parents in distress. These services may reduce anxiety, detect health problems early and occasionally may even avert death.

Only a few of the schemes described have been subjected to any form of evaluation. However several lessons appear to have been learnt. Perhaps the most important is that if such services are to be established with any permanence, careful attention must be given to the needs of the professionals concerned: their pay, workload, hours of work, safety, and the organisation of their own family life. It is hard to escape the conclusion that it is short-sighted to leave the development of such innovatory services to altruism alone. These schemes do not cost much, but their future probably depends on the availability of *some* extra resources, particularly more midwives and health visitors.

Notes

1   Miss R. Craven, Senior Nursing Officer (Midwifery), Royal Shrewsbury Hospital (Maternity), Mutton Oak Road, Copthorne, Shrewsbury SY3 BXF
2   Miss I. Waterhouse, Divisional Nursing Officer (Midwifery and Gynaecology), W. Berkshire HA, 3 Craven Road, Reading RG1 5LF, Berks
3   Director of Nursing Services (Community), Huddersfield Health Authority, Civic Centre, High Street, Huddersfield, West Yorkshire
4   Miss M. Haylock, Senior Nursing Officer, Enfield Health Authority, 100 Church Street, Enfield, Middlesex EN2 6PS
5   Director of Nursing Services (Community), N. E. Essex Health Authority, East Lodge Court, High Street, Colchester CO1 1UJ
6   Divisional Nursing Officer (Community), Harrow Hospital, Roxeth Hill, Harrow, Middlesex HA2 0JX
7   Mrs A. Bogie, Nursing Officer, Ham Clinic, Ham Drive, Plymouth, Devon
8   Director of Nursing Services (Community), Kingston and Esher Health Authority, 17 Upper Brighton Road, Surbiton, Surrey KT6 6LH
9   Director of Nursing Services (Community), Barnet HA, Telford House, Woodside Lane, London N1 28RL

6 Health and the education services

So far the focus has been mainly on schemes in which health service staff are trying to make the NHS more attractive and accessible to all parents, in pregnancy and during children's early years. But the achievement of a genuinely preventive health care system will entail drawing on resources outside the NHS, central and essential though that is. Information and education, social support and care, adequate income and housing, self-esteem and control over one's own life are some of the crucial ingredients for health.

During my research, listening to people talk about their work, it has become increasingly clear that a surprising range of agencies outside the NHS see themselves in this business of health care. I have heard from teachers, social workers, housing officers, volunteers, pharmacists, trade unions, employers and many others. The message of their evidence is powerful. Health in pregnancy and early childhood is not the sole concern of the health professions or the NHS. It follows, therefore, that the resources for health and health care should not be seen within these narrow confines.

Such sentiments are not new. They are in accord with the government's health policies, as well as with those of WHO. Health professionals are urged to recognise the range of agencies in the community concerned with health and to develop ways of working with them (DHSS 1981a and c; WHO 1981).

But the difficulties of moving from the rhetoric of policy statements to operational change should not be underestimated. If health promotion schemes in the community are to be developed further, within each agency concerned there must be motivation for change, as well as the necessary resources and skills for new developments. At a time of economic recession, with government policies set on reducing public sector spending, it is hard to see how these criteria will be met. Many health authorities are experiencing zero or negative growth in their services; local authority departments are suffering severe cuts in their budgets; voluntary organisations, too, are feeling the effects of the recession. When services are fighting hard for their very survival, new developments and collaborative ventures between different sectors of care will be difficult to achieve.

But despite these problems, there are likely to be many real or potential community resources for health in every neighbourhood:

some of them probably unknown or unrecognised by health authorities and their staff. Their assistance is needed for the prevention of ill-health. Though at present it is hard to find funds for their support, the new arrangements for Joint Finance[1] may be important in this respect; so too may be special grants from central government for community projects.

This chapter and chapters 7 and 8 describe schemes relevant to family health coming from the education services, the personal social services, and from volunteers and voluntary organisations respectively. Chapter 9 illustrates ways in which health service staff can work with these different agencies to facilitate a greater range and volume of community resources for family health.

Schemes are described in this chapter which come from local education authority primary and secondary schools as well as the various providers of adult education. Most of the schemes can be broadly classified as concerned with health education and, in particular, education and support for pregnancy and early child care and development. These are important aspects of preventive health care, yet ones to which most health professionals can give little time, resources or trained expertise. Health education officers and health visitors are probably the exception. But even they may not be equipped to meet the complex educational needs of some of the most educationally and socially disadvantaged children and families: the very people who may be most in need of them.

Children in school are important audiences for courses in education for parenthood. The first part of this chapter refers briefly to these. But captive audiences should not be equated with captive minds. Education for parenthood points to futures which may seem unrealistic and remote to many schoolchildren. There is a need for education services which reach out to adults, at times when such learning is most immediately relevant. For the present study, this means during pregnancy and the earliest years of parenting and childhood. The second part of this chapter describes three such schemes which have developed from adult education. These are particularly relevant to this study as they illustrate strategies to try and reverse the 'Inverse Care Law' (Tudor Hart, J. 1971) as it applies to adult education. Its implication is that those with the greatest need for further learning opportunities are the least likely to achieve access to them.

The final project described in this chapter is perhaps the most unusual, and for me the most exciting. It indicates that children's learning programmes can provide a new type of resource for health and development extending to families in communities around schools. Also it implies that we may deny ourselves important avenues of caring by placing schoolchildren in the role of passive receivers, rather than active contributors to community services.

Health and parenthood studies for children in schools

Teachers, health visitors, midwives and health education officers stressed the importance of courses in schools on health in parenthood and early child development.

> If there is a real interest in reaching the consumer with information for health, what better place to catch them than the classroom? After all, this is about the only place where we can be sure of contacting virtually *every* future parent. We shouldn't waste the opportunity. (A health visitor)

The variety of approaches in school programmes to education for parenthood is reflected in their titles: 'child care', 'child development', 'preparation for family life', 'citizenship courses', 'social education' and 'health education'. Most of these courses cover some aspects of health care during pregnancy and childhood and refer to the importance of attending clinics regularly. A few are trying to increase children's confidence in their own abilities to seek assistance from services which may seem bewilderingly complex.

While collecting material for the study I have talked to teachers, HM Inspectors of Schools and others concerned with these types of educational programmes. From these discussions several common themes emerged about ways which may make such learning attractive and interesting for schoolchildren.[2] As these aspects of the teaching/learning process are relevant to this study of 'ways of reaching the consumer', they are briefly summarised below. For more detailed information about the different approaches used in 'preparation for parenthood' courses, readers are referred to the National Children's Bureau's study, 'Preparation and Support for Parents with Young Children' (Pugh, G. 1980).

1 In many schools it seems that education for parenthood is still seen as an exclusively female subject and one which is of secondary importance to academic achievement. However, a few schools have made such courses compulsory for all boys and girls. Some voluntary courses succeed in attracting boys, possibly because attention has been given to making their contents and titles attractive and relevant to their interests as young men.

2 The subject does not seem to lend itself to didactic teaching styles. Indeed, it is one in which there are few universally 'right' choices. Individuals can only be guided towards informed

and rational choices appropriate to their own worlds. The difficulties of such an approach for teachers, or anyone else involved, should not be underestimated. It runs counter to much of their training and experience; it also assumes that they are not inhibited by their own values and their own sexuality.

3 It seems important to link the specialist teaching skills of teachers with the information and resource facilities of health professionals and the health service. Some schools' schemes work in close co-operation with local health visitors, GPs and health education officers.

4 Teaching programmes which enable children to take an active and responsible role in learning appear to be popular. Children may visit clinics, talk to health visitors, midwives and doctors, help the clinic nurse and have opportunities to talk with mothers in small groups. Secondary schoolchildren have carried out special projects, learning about pregnancy and early child care by being 'attached' to local mothers both during their pregnancies and the babies' first few months of life. They may sometimes accompany them on their visits to clinics. Some school courses also give children the opportunity of working in playgroups and nurseries. Here, their direct involvement with young children teaches them about the different stages of early child development.

Such 'learning by doing' programmes seem to be more demanding of teaching and support staff than classroom-based courses. They require much planning and collaboration with the agencies to which the children go. Those involved in such schemes emphasise that children should be adequately prepared for their visits so that they know the type of information they should acquire and the observations which they should make. Supervision and support during learning are also important.

Those responsible for finding suitable placements should beware of overloading the receiving organisation. The staff of clinics and playgroups should not be prevented from carrying out their legitimate function. The number of places available is often, therefore, limited.

Health and parenthood studies for adults

Learning does not have to be confined to classrooms at prescribed and sometimes inappropriate times of life. The adult education services[3] provide ways by which people can return to learning opportunities after their schooldays as and when they feel them necessary. The next three schemes have been chosen to show the

variety of approaches which are used to make health and parenthood studies attractive and accessible for parents. They are
particularly concerned with those whom the education services
sometimes fail to reach effectively: ethnic minorities, and people
living in difficult and impoverished conditions.

*HELP, Leeds, an English-as-a-second-language maternity language
project*

In parts of the country where large proportions of births are in
communities where little English is spoken, some English-as-a-
second-language (ESL) courses now focus on the language needs of
pregnant mothers and of families with young children. They aim
to help their students to use the health services more confidently
and appropriately while also imparting some basic health education. The maternity language course at the Harehills English
Language Project (HELP)[4] in Leeds is an example of such a
scheme.

HELP began in 1976 as part of the job creation scheme, but was
soon adopted by Leeds Local Education Authority's continuing
education programme. Five full-time and several part-time workers
were employed to teach English to members of all ethnic groups,
the majority in Leeds being Punjabis from Pakistan and India, and
Bangladeshis. The project offered a wide range of courses
including some on health topics.

The teachers soon realised that many of the Asian women
students had difficulty in understanding the specialised medical
terminology of pregnancy and childbirth and thus could not make
the best use of the health services during this crucial time.
Difficulties arose when trying to communicate their health
problems to midwives and doctors, as well as when attempting to
follow their instructions and to complete the necessary forms.
The teachers found it difficult to introduce the subjects of
pregnancy and childbirth into the normal language classes, as there
was a natural shyness and reticence in the group. It was decided,
therefore, to design a separate course for pregnant women and
women with young children.

Early in 1977, with the help of midwives, health visitors and
doctors, the project teachers started to devise their new course,
known as the Maternity Language Course. It was tested and
modified with some sixty Asian students over a total of six courses
spread over two years.

The final version of the teaching material has been published,
together with detailed instructions so that it can be used by
people with little or no teaching experience.[5] It consists of
twenty units which can be used with individuals or small groups.
It is structured on the assumption that women will start attending

the classes between the third and eighth month of pregnancy, that many of them will not be used to formalised learning and that they will be unlikely to attend every class.

Emphasis has been placed on the visual demonstration of information by pictures and by role play. The course starts with the language mothers will encounter when their history is taken at the first booking-clinic, explaining the reasons for certain types of examinations and tests and what these involve, stressing the importance of continuing health and dental care, good diet and nutrition. The course then leads on to the language needed to understand and be involved in hospital routine and the birth of the baby. It ends with topics such as infant feeding, the needs of the new baby at home and the importance of postnatal care and family planning. It also includes information on welfare rights in pregnancy and the postnatal period.

The introduction of preventive health care programmes like HELP provide a useful opportunity to monitor the effect of such interventions on health behaviour (have the number of parents and children attending clinics increased?) and also health information and language. With the limited resources available, this has not been possible in HELP. However, when asked about the effectiveness of the teaching programme, the course tutor emphasised the difficulty of assessing the small gains which may be made in only a few teaching sessions by women who understand and read no English. Her subjective impression of their success was that although few women have developed much fluent expressive language as a result of the course, many of them have improved their comprehension. Perhaps more importantly, the tutor thought there had been a gradual spread of information concerning antenatal and child care from the groups of students to their relatives and friends.

The Open University's parent and health education courses

The Open University (OU) is well known for its undergraduate programmes, which offer adults the opportunity to study for a degree at home in their spare time. Their community education section[6] designs short practical courses aimed at the community at large, rather than only those wanting a degree. In the field of parent and health education they have devised a variety of strategies to try and remove the barriers which may hold back those least likely to take up further learning opportunities. Their work is therefore relevant to this study. It is also remarkable for the way in which the course material has been made so widely available to health visitors, midwives and GPs. For these reasons it seems appropriate to describe the development of two of these courses in some detail: 'The First Years of Life' (covering the ages from birth to three years)[7] and 'The Pre-School Child' (covering the ages from three to five years).

In their basic form, each of these courses lasts eight weeks and consists of printed material, TV and radio programmes, and a resource pack containing cassettes, records, study guides, quizzes and computer-marked assignments.

Self-help discussion groups To help the students get the most out of these materials, the OU has encouraged the formation of local self-help discussion groups. Members of the Pre-school Play-group Association as well as some health education officers and health visitors have played an important part in establishing these groups. It was hoped that the involvement of these key community workers would attract parents with few or no previous educational qualifications into the courses (Calder, J. and Lilley, A. 1978a and b).

Like many health education schemes, however, the OU course was not entirely successful in attracting this type of parent. Analysis of the educational profiles of 'The First Year of Life' students showed that they differed little from those taking the standard OU undergraduate programmes. The unusual feature of the OU story, however, has been that they have not accepted this situation, but have devised new strategies to make these courses more widely available.

The Free Place scheme For instance, the Free Place scheme provides free places for low-income parents (Sheilds, J. 1979). Health visitors and others working in the community identify and encourage the free enrolment of those most likely to benefit from these courses.[8] In 1978/79, the first year of the scheme, the Health Education Council sponsored 1,000 such free places. By 1981/82 this number had quadrupled. The evaluation of the scheme suggests that this approach has succeeded in increasing the recruitment of students who have few or no educational qualifications.

Course extracts without course registration Some parents may be deterred from joining the courses by the form-filling procedures which are required for enrolment. To try and overcome this problem the OU has encouraged the use of their course materials wherever they may be helpful, irrespective of course registration. The Health Education Council has funded the printing costs of some 50,000 leaflets containing extracts from 'The First Years of Life' and 'The Pre-School Child'. These have been used by health visitors, midwives and others working with individuals and groups such as antenatal classes, postnatal and mother-and-toddler groups

(Calder, J. *et al.* 1979; Chapman, S. and Reynolds, E. 1982; Palfreeman, S. 1982).

The evaluation of the use of the HEC leaflets, as well as the Free Place scheme, has highlighted the importance of personal support and encouragement in learning, particularly for the most socially and educationally disadvantaged parents. Health visitors, health education officers and other community workers can only spare a limited amount of time to provide such support. The OU has therefore looked for modifications to the way the materials are used so that less individual learning support is needed.

Working with local radio and press   In 1979 this became possible when joint projects were set up between the OU and commercial local radio stations in Bradford and Birmingham. The OU prepared a special fifteen-page booklet with modified material from the 'Pre-School Child' course. Listeners were offered this booklet free. Additional learning support came from the local radio stations, each of which independently produced a series of relevant programmes. One of the stations broadcast these over a six-week period and timed them to coincide with the publication of printed extracts from the original course in the local newspaper.

From the data available on learners' participation in these radio schemes, it appears that they attracted a wide ability range, including more than expected with minimal educational qualifications. On criteria such as the courses' 'interest' and 'usefulness' and the learners' 'satisfactions', no difference was found between those classified as high- and low-ability learners (Lilley, A. 1980).

'The Book of the Child'   The Scottish Health Education Unit has also modified the OU's course material so that it can be used with little additional learning support. With extensive research and testing, topics from 'The First Years of Life' and 'The Pre-School Child' have been presented in a booklet entitled 'The Book of the Child' (1980). The language and layout have been designed to be attractive and easy to use by parents at the lower end of the reading-ability scale. This booklet is being distributed free by midwives and health visitors to every pregnant woman in Scotland. At the time of writing at least one health authority in England has funded a special printing of this booklet for all their parents, with their own cover and list of 'useful addresses' to make it look local. In 1981 the cost of this was 50 pence per copy.

Starting again with parents' needs   In the development of learning materials described so far, the staff of the OU have decided which are the issues appropriate to include in the courses. They have also devised the structure of the learning material. The

experience of many community teachers in socially disadvantaged communities suggests that this approach may be counter-
productive. It may offer learning which is not directly relevant to
people's everyday problems (Fordham, P. *et al.* 1979; Hubley, J.
and Sheldon, H. 1980). Put simply, to cope with the health and
development of their children, parents first have to cope with their
own problems.

With these observations in mind the OU has established a special
research project funded by the Bernard Van Leer Foundation. It
aims to find ways in which learners themselves can determine the
content of their learning. The project includes groups of mothers
in run-down areas in Birmingham, Liverpool, Coventry and in
isolated communities of the Western Isles. The project staff
concentrate on identifying these parents' worries about bringing
up their children and the way in which these are dealt with in
group discussions. This work shows that in these groups parenting
tends to be seen in the context of everyday difficulties, such as
poor housing, loneliness and low incomes. These subjects then
provide the basic topics around which the project team develop
new and relevant learning materials. This is done by combining
the expertise and resources of the OU with the experience of the
local groups.

In summary, this is a story which highlights many of the features
important in modifying standard services to reach people who
would probably otherwise not use them. It is a story of trial and
error, of great flexibility in ways of working and of generous and
imaginative attempts at experimentation. Central to these developments has been the discipline of the continuous process of
defining the works' objectives, stating hypotheses about the
possible ways of achieving them, evaluating and recording their
validity and then modifying the original approach. In all this work
the range of agencies in the community with which the OU has
worked has been impressive and demonstrates the importance of
working through many different channels and across many
different service barriers to attract the people who are least likely
to take up further learning opportunities.

*Educational home visiting: the ILEA's south-east London home
visiting scheme*

The last of the three adult education projects which I will describe
comes from educational home visiting, a movement which origin-
ated in the USA in the 1960s. A decade later it developed in this
country, stimulated by the Plowden Report on Primary Education
(Central Advisory Council for Education 1967). This recommended an expansion of nursery education, particulary for
children living in socially disadvantaged areas.

Educational home-visiting schemes have developed a variety of strategies which combine pre-school and adult educational skills and resources with social support and liaison work with other agencies (Aplin, G. and Pugh, G. 1983). Teachers and others with suitable training reach isolated, depressed and disadvantaged families and young children in their homes. Research suggests that their intervention may have a positive effect on these children's development (Lazar, F. *et al.* 1977; Weikat, D. *et al.* 1978). It probably also contributes to the parents' feeling of self-confidence and promotes their interest and involvement in their children's learning (Armstrong, G. and Brown, F. 1979). Educational home visiting, therefore, may be an important service for the promotion of such families' health and development. It can provide a form of preventive care which, by the nature of things, is beyond the scope of the NHS.

In 1973 the publication of the ILEA's document 'An Education Service for the Whole Community' marked a new phase in their educational policy. Teachers were encouraged to take their skills out of the classrooms into the community to try and reach the children and families who made least use of the educational services available. In 1974, in response to this, the principal of the Frobisher Adult Education Institute (now the Southwark Institute of Adult Education[9]) and the headmistress of Clyde Nursery School initiated the Deptford Educational Home Visiting Scheme.

Objectives   The objectives and design of the project were formulated with the involvement of the staff of the two local health centres, Lewisham Social Services Department, representatives from the Community Relations Council and the Research and Statistics Group of the ILEA.

By visiting homes, the project hopes to reach parents who traditionally feel the child's education starts only when he enters school and who are unaware of the importance of their own role in the early development of their children. We hope that by helping parents to develop and reinforce their skills as educators, their children will be enabled to have greater opportunities to achieve their full potential.

(ILEA Educational Home Visiting Project 1977)

Staff and training   At the start of the project a full-time co-ordinator and five educational home visitors were appointed to the staff of the Frobisher Adult Education Institute. Only one of the home visitors was a trained teacher. The others were playgroup and play-scheme supervisors and a social studies diploma student. Their initial three weeks' training included sessions with health visitors, social workers and community workers. They covered topics such as language development, the role of play in cognitive and language development, the special problems associated with adult learning and how to keep records.

EHVs' work At the start of the Deptford project, educational home visiting was offered to all parents with 2-year-olds born in a certain six-month period who were on the lists of two local health centres. Initial contact was made by their health visitor or the headmistress of the nursery school. No attempt was made at this stage to favour families who had particular problems with their children, as project workers feared that educational home visiting might be seen as a stigma of bad parenting. In the first year, thirty-two families with a child of about two years old were visited weekly. In the second year this figure almost doubled. At this time the visitors, working part-time, could each cope with twelve to fifteen visits a week.

Each visitor had access to toys and books which she could take into the home for play with the children which could involve the mothers. The emphasis in the first visits was on the building of trust and acceptance between the family and the home visitor. Whenever possible mothers and fathers were involved in planning the weekly play sessions, to which children generally responded enthusiastically. Mothers often expressed surprise at the achievement and knowledge which the sessions revealed in their children. But for these mothers themselves there were frequent problems of depression, poverty and exhaustion from overwork. As time went on the home visitors found themselves increasingly involved in supporting and caring for the mothers, and this enabled them, in turn, to support the children. A programme of group activities for parents was set up in easily accessible places, which proved so popular that it developed into informal adult education sessions that covered different topics such as keeping fit, cookery and toy-making.

The results of the ILEA's monitoring programme carried out during the first year of the project were encouraging. Though based on a small sample, it suggested that children who were visited might have better language comprehension than that of a control group of children not visited. Their parents also had a greater interest in being involved in their children's education (Jayne, E. 1976).

At the end of the second year the project team were so convinced of the importance of their work they felt it should be extended to other parts of south-east London, but unfortunately, no further resources were available. They therefore decided to reduce their staff of educational home visitors in Deptford from

four to one.   The other three each moved to set up a similar
project in a new area.   As there was now only one home visitor
working in each area, new ways of increasing their contact with
families had to be found.   They set up mother-and-toddler groups
and, in one area, volunteer home visitors were trained to work
under the supervision of the paid educational home visitor.

Health visitors' involvement   Health visitors have been quick to
appreciate that this new development can supplement their own
limited home-visiting resources. Educational home visitors increase
the help available for some of the most isolated and depressed
families in the neighbourhood, who may require skilled educational
and supportive work.   Local health visitors now work closely with
the project, referring families for educational home visiting,
assisting in visitors' training sessions and giving talks and joining in
parents' group meetings.   In one area, the educational home
visiting team has been invited to hold its group meetings for
parents and children in the nearby health centre.   The nursing
officer wrote:

> The toddler groups held at the Bermondsey health centre
> provide a service which is much appreciated by health visitors
> working in the area. It is often possible for a young mother not
> to know her nearest neighbour and until her child is three and
> can go to nursery, there is no formal provision for socialisation
> . . . mothers who have been sceptical about the value of play
> and appropriate toys, about reading to their toddler and even
> talking to them are converted by the example of the EHV and
> of other mothers.   (ILEA 1979)

Development of other schemes   Since the start of educational
home visiting in the early 1970s, other schemes have developed
throughout the country.   Some of these have been funded by
LEAs, others depend on voluntary funding and volunteer home
visitors.   The emphasis on parent support and education has
tended to increase.   It is now recognised that for many educationally and socially disadvantaged families, assistance in dealing with
the parents' own lives can have an important effect on their
childrens' development (Aplin, G. and Pugh, G. 1983).   This
changing focus from early child to adult education is well illustrated
by the Homelink Scheme in Liverpool (one of the local groups in
the OU's Bernard Van Leer project — see page 75), and in Scope,
Southampton. The latter scheme is described in chapter 9.

School children as a health resource in the community

In the next project, the resources for health come from schools rather than from adult education institutions. It is the children and the disabled, usually cast in the role of passive service receivers, who are the inspiration behind these resources. This blurring of the distinction between active 'givers' and passive 'receivers' in education is reminiscent of the participation processes which are described in health care schemes in chapter 10. As in these schemes, it seems that active participation has liberated ideas and energies for community care. Teachers and other adults, not previously aware of this enormous potential, have been surprised at what has developed.

It would be misleading, however, to suggest that this type of programme, with redefined roles for teachers, health professionals, children and disabled people, are easy or cheap to establish. The following description indicates the extraordinary amount of energy, time and commitment which has to be devoted to setting up, maintaining and supporting them. It also hints at the type of people who may be needed to establish such ways of working: good communicators, people with a wide knowledge of the different community agencies, workers who can quickly establish trust and who are flexible in their work and prepared to take some risks.

CSV's School Concern Project, Salford

The School Concern Project[10] began in 1979 as a joint venture between Community Service Volunteers (CSV),[11] Salford Education Authority and Salford Social Services Department. In two years, with a grant from the DHSS, its team has shown how the resources of primary schools through to sixth form colleges can be harnessed to design, invent and make devices which disabled people need to manage their daily lives. Most of these aids have been for adults and other children, but some have been for the under-fives and their parents. It seems likely that this age pattern reflects only the project's main source of referrals and not the need for this type of assistance in the younger age groups. Because of the potential of this type of scheme for working with disabled parents and very young children, perhaps identified by health visitors, GPs or paediatricians, it is described in some detail.

The advisory group and project team　At the start of the project CSV were careful to engage the interest and commitment of the senior managers of the key statutory agencies who would be involved. This proved a crucial factor in the success of their work. An advisory group was established, composed of senior officers from the local authority departments of education and social services and the CSV. They helped to start the scheme, appointed the professional team members, and provided them with advice and support.

The members of the project team were selected to provide a range of professional expertise which complemented that already available in the schools. There was a co-ordinator, an occupational therapist, a writer/researcher, a craft/design teacher and up to eight full-time community service volunteers. The skilled and practical assistance which this team could offer teachers seems to have been important in establishing schools' confidence in working with the project. The team's base was in a local teachers' centre which, together with secretarial and office support, was provided free of charge by the LEA.

Involvement with schools   The team's first task was to foster links between the schools and the agencies which put them in touch with disabled people. These were mainly people working in special schools, daycentres and residential centres. Practical problems also needed careful attention: transport to bring the children and disabled people together, special insurance to cover the pupils when working outside their schools, sources of materials for the aids and adequate workshop space.

Time was given to talking about the project with everyone who would be involved in its work in the schools. Their fears as well as their ideas were listened to. It was quickly recognised that considerable preparation of the staff as well as the children was needed before they started working with disabled people. The disabled also needed preparation to know how much they could expect from their young colleagues. The project team therefore collated and designed learning materials on disability as well as on many other aspects of their work.

The following account describes the project's work with a primary school. The report of the Salford scheme gives many examples which involve secondary school children (CSV 1981):

> When first approached by members of the project team the Head and the Deputy Head of St John's C. of E. Primary School were cautious. They were concerned that their pupils would not be able to meet the demands — emotional and technical — they thought would be required of them. Eventually, however, after much discussion with the staff, a small group of the upper juniors was chosen to work on aid-making, and links were quickly established between St John's and a school for ESN(S) children . . .
> Children from the Special School and St John's School began

to exchange visits on a regular basis, each becoming involved in the general routine of the other's school. In this way the St John's children quickly learned from the ESN(S) children about the nature of their disabilities and the sort of problems these created for them in everyday life. They were then able to work with them to design appropriate aides. For instance they saw their difficulties in co-ordinating their movements. Tasks such as dressing, which the St John's children did with ease, could be frustrating and laborious for the pupils of the special school. They therefore designed a simple aid to help them master the art of fastening buttons and zipping zippers.

BUTTONING EXCERCISES
First take a normal shirt and sew it all up, leaving a small
(but not too small) hole. Add stuffing until the shirt is
plump. The buttons can then be fastened and unfastened.
Children who have difficulty picking up or using small
items will be able to practice on the shirts you make.
You could add zips or other buttons to give more practice.

The project co-ordinator described the process of designing and making aids as 'one of trial and error, which allowed the children to discover their mistakes themselves. As their skills improved, so their confidence grew — they became inventors.' The gain was for the schools too. Craftwork took on a new meaning as children who had previously been busy with pipe-racks and flowerpot holders found that their skills and ideas were in real demand.

The role of the project team in all this work was that of a resource and facilitating agent. Once schools were linked with disabled people, and teachers were familiar with the knowledge they required and were confident in their abilities to work in this field, the team could withdraw, but continued to provide an advice service for the teachers whenever this was needed.

This pattern of a large injection of skills and resources at the start of a school's work, followed by the gradual and planned withdrawal of the team's direct involvement, was probably important in enabling teachers and children to realise their own abilities. It helped to ensure that schools did not become too dependent on the short-lived project team.

As the end of the two-year grant approached the team concentrated on incorporating the information they had gathered into learning materials. They also helped establish a local support group of people interested in the schools' work, which gradually took over the CSV teams' work, offering practical assistance and advice to schools when needed. The group consists of teachers, occupational therapists, social workers and disabled people.

Spreading the scheme beyond Salford   A particularly impressive aspect of all CSV's work is their emphasis on the documentation of projects and the dissemination of their findings and ways of working. This is made possible through the national organisation of CSV which provides specialist advice and resources for the development of printed materials. Through their media unit they also assist local projects in working with TV, radio and the press.

With this support the Salford team have been able to make the experience of their small local project available to a national and even international audience. During the two years of their funding they produced a written report describing the development of their project in detail, together with a 'Starters' Pack' for teachers, giving the information and material needed to set up similar projects.[12] They also made videos, tape/slide sets and audio cassettes on various aspects of their work. The project received extensive publicity through the local and national media. This resulted in over 500 enquiries from individuals and local authorities wanting to set up similar schemes. Considerable interest has also been shown overseas, for instance in Sweden, Norway, the USA and Japan.

Though the CSV team in Salford has now been disbanded, its original co-ordinator was funded for a limited period to continue to disseminate their work more widely. If requested he would visit an area, hold discussions with interested groups and advise on possible developments.

The scheme and general practice   Perhaps because the project is still little known in medical circles, I could only find one GP (in North Humberside) who has responded to the potential of the scheme for the health service.[13] He heard the Salford co-ordinator speaking about his work on a radio programme and quickly contacted him for further details. Within a few months he had persuaded the head of his local comprehensive school and the LEA's advisor for craft and design technology to establish a similar project in liaison with his practice. Writing about his ideas for the future of this scheme he commented:

> I think it is preferable for the school children to see the disabled person in his or her own house if this can be arranged, rather than attendance at local authority clinics or day centres, which in fact contain only a small proportion of the total disabled . . . Written consent of participation is preferable provided that the patient can write. Parents consent should be obtained in cases under school leaving age or of mental subnormality.
>
> I am not sure to what extent professionals should interfere with the assessment of disability made by the pupils; part of

the learning process after all . . . We may be surprised that the pupil discovers some aspect of the disability that we have missed.

Such schemes would seem to have an exciting potential for the health care of all age groups in the community, including disabled parents and very young children. So far, the failure of the scheme to be taken up by GPs and health visitors is in marked contrast to its success with local authority departments and schools. This probably reflects only the project's focus on contacting disabled people through institutional settings, for example daycentres, special schools. There is a need now to direct publicity about the scheme to primary health care workers, particularly GPs and community nurses.

In conclusion

This chapter highlights the place of the educational services in the future development of family health care. Parents should have basic information about the causes of health and ill-health. They need to understand the way their children develop from conception to adulthood, how this development can best be supported and how they can cope with the realities of being parents. They should also know what financial benefits they are entitled to. These may help parents provide children with a safer and less stressful environment. They have a right to know how to use the NHS for the prevention as well as the cure of diseases.

The skills and resources of the educational services are needed to complement those of health authorities and general practitioners in meeting these requirements. Basic training programmes, as well as later in-service courses for health professionals, should give information about relevant educational developments and services. The government should consider urgently ways of promoting the use of Joint Finance (from health authority budgets) by local authorities.[14] It should be used imaginatively to develop collaborative health and education schemes which will improve the delivery of health information and care.

Notes

1 Joint Finance comes from the NHS expenditure and is intended to assist collaboration between health and local authority services in areas of common concern. For further details concerning your own health authority contact the district health authority administrator. (See also note 14.)
2 At the time of writing aspects of the secondary school curriculum relating to education for parenthood are being evaluated by Professor R. Whitfield, Aston University, Birmingham.

3 Adult education is mainly concerned with non-vocational, non-professional and non-qualification courses, these usually being part-time. Important providers of AE are local education authorities, university extra-mural departments, the Workers' Education Association and the Open University. See *The Year Book of Adult Education* published by The National Institute of Adult Education, for names and addresses of AE establishments in each local authority area.

4 HELP, Leeds Adult Literary Department, 27 Harrogate Road, Leeds 7

5 Available from the Printed Resources Unit for Continuing Education, 27 Harrogate Road, Leeds 7.
Some other sources of antenatal and child health ESL teaching materials are:

   1 Your health authority's health education officer.

   2 The Commission for Racial Equality, Elliot House, 10/11 Allington Street, London SW1E 5EH ('Antenatal Language Kit')

   3 Milton Keynes Voluntary Language Scheme, The Queensway Centre, The Queensway, Bletchley, Milton Keynes MK2 2HB ('The New Baby' and 'Taking Care of the Family')

   4 Language Development Unit, Floor B, Great Moore Street, Bolton, BL1 1NS ('Appointment at the Antenatal Clinic').

   5 The National Extension College, 18 Brooklands Avenue, Cambridge ('Zorina Begum Thinks She Is Pregnant', 'Communicating with the System' — A workbook on Health Services' and 'Mother and Baby Care: a pack for tutors and students of English as a second language').

   6 Bolton Road Centre for Language and Literacy, Manningham, Bradford 8 ('Booking in at the Antenatal Clinic', 'Mrs Worth has a Baby' and 'Bottlefeeding', also 'Sakira goes to the Antenatal Clinic' and 'Sakira goes into Hospital'.

   7 National Association for the Teaching of English as a Second Language for Adults (NATESLA), 59 Station Road, Codsall, Wolverhampton WV8 1BY. Regional branches may assist local projects.

6 Centre for Continuing Education, The Open University, PO Box 188, Sherwood House, Bletchley, Milton Keynes MK3 6HW

7 A restructured version of this course is being prepared for 1983/84. Other courses in this series include 'Childhood Five to Ten', 'Adolescence' and 'Health Choices'.

8 For details of this scheme, write to The Open University. (See note 6.)

9 Mary Marsh, EHV Co-ordinator, Southwark Institute of Adult Education, St Mary's Road, London SE15 2EA

10 Disabled Resources Information Service, Salford Resource Centre, Hyde Lodge, Half Edge Lane, Eccles, Manchester M30 9GD

11 CSV is the British counterpart of 'Voluntary Service Overseas' (VSO). It is a voluntary organisation giving opportunities for community voluntary service in this country rather than overseas.

12 Available from CSV, 237 Pentonville Road, London, N1 9NJ.

13 Dr J. Keel, 36 West End, South Cave, Brough HU15 2EY

14 At the time of writing, Joint Finance from the NHS is only available to schemes for a limited number of years. Local authorities must then take on the funding. At present Joint Finance schemes are included in local authority budgets and therefore makes them more likely to face rate support grant penalties for overspending their budgetry targets.

7 Health and the personal social services

The subject of this chapter is the personal social services and the relevance of their resources and skills to health in pregnancy and early childhood.

Social services departments have a responsibility for meeting the social needs of certain children and their families, especially those who have physical and mental disabilities, those living in poverty and in deprived environments and those experiencing disturbed family relationships. These responsibilities are met in a variety of ways. Social workers provide practical advice and information on matters such as income and housing, and they have a range of special skills and the training needed to help families with complex and problematic personal relationships. The departments provide residential services, day nurseries and domiciliary services such as home helps, laundry services and the fitting of aids and adaptions for the homes of disabled children and parents. Social services departments also supervise privately run playgroups and childminders in their areas.

With these resources and skills, the departments have an important role to play in promoting health in pregnancy and early childhood. They can positively influence some of the key factors which are associated with patterns of ill-health, particularly in families living in stressful and impoverishing circumstances. For instance, a social worker who is well informed about welfare rights may encourage a new mother on supplementary benefit to apply for single payments for equipment, such as a new sterilisation unit, extra heaters and a safe cot. Relatively small investments in social care in pregnancy and early childhood, particularly for families with unusually stressful lives, might result in long-term savings for the health and social services.

At another level, also, social services departments are important in preventive health care. Those working in them are often in contact with the very families who the preventive health services find difficult to reach, and may have the skills to maintain contact with them when other agencies fail. These elusive families are often the parents and children who are most in need of health information and care. This point was recognised in the Short Report on Perinatal and Neonatal Mortality (1980) and the Court Report on the Child Health Services (1976). Social services' personnel can link parents and children to midwives, health visitors and other appropriate sources of health care. Sometimes they may themselves provide the information and care needed, ideally with the advice of a health professional.

The schemes described in this chapter illustrate these different aspects of health promotion. It must be stressed, however, that they represent only a tiny fraction of the work of these departments in promoting the health of parents and children.

Avon's Home Aide Scheme

Avon's Home Aide Scheme[1] shows how the home care services (including home helps and home aides) can act as bridging agents between the health services and families by providing information and care for health. It is also an example of the way in which resources can be redefined to meet new needs.

The increasing numbers of old people within Avon's population are making extensive demands on all the health and social services. In 1977 the social services department responded to this by enlarging their home care team to include trained and specialised home aides as well as home helps. This new development brings together some of the skills of nursing, social work and teaching as well as the practical domestic skills of home helps. Its objective is to provide an intensive support service for individuals in their own homes in situations which might otherwise break down and require admission to hospital or residential care.

Although the elderly provide the majority of the schemes' cases, families with young children and women experiencing difficult pregnancies are also included. For acceptance into the scheme all referrals have to be made with the agreement of the full clinical and social work team concerned. There also has to be a strong likelihood that the service will be needed for no more than six weeks. In the three-month period from April to June 1980, the four area teams received a total of two hundred and six new referrals, of which one hundred and forty-two (69 per cent) were accepted. Just under half the rejected referrals were described as inappropriate for the type of service offered. Most of the remainder were turned down due to a shortage of home aides.

Home aides are chosen for their previous experience and training, notably as nurses, social work assistants or teachers. Upon appointment they receive two weeks' intensive training in both the health and social services. This includes work in hospitals and is followed at intervals by further relevant training.

At the start of the scheme in 1977 there were ten aides, each working an eight-hour rota for five days in every seven. Since then, the service has gradually expanded, so that by 1980 there were fifty aides, divided into four area teams. In 1983, the number had increased to sixty-five, with the addition of an extra area team. The work of each team is co-ordinated by a qualified Home Aide Organiser. The cost of the scheme in 1978/79 was £40,000, rising to £86,000 in 1982/83. It is jointly financed by the health authority and county council. No charge is made to the recipients of its services.

The case of an unsupported mother returning home to her 3-year-old son with her newborn triplets provides an example of the complex problems which this service is prepared to tackle. It also shows how home aides' work is designed to increase people's independence, rather than to make them dependent on their services. Such ways of working demand much support and resources at the start, when those receiving the service have little confidence in their own abilities. As confidence grows, so the home aides' support is lessened and gradually withdrawn.

Mrs X was a single mother with four children — a 3-year-old, and new-born triplets. She had an obsessional illness, causing her to wash herself and the children repeatedly. She disliked her social worker who she thought would take the children into care. Relationships with her health visitor were little better.

Before Mrs X was discharged from hospital, the home aide organiser met with all the key members of the health and social work team involved to agree a plan of care. An aide visited Mrs X before she left hospital and was quickly accepted as a friend. Once Mrs X was home, the aide spent eight hours a day with the family, establishing a routine for the babies, helping the mother feed, change and bath them.

According to the agreed plan, the health visitor and social worker visited the family infrequently. However they kept in close contact with the home aide, giving her whatever advice she needed. The aide had frequent meetings and contact with her home aide organiser. As with all cases, she kept notes of each day's activities, progress and problems and prepared weekly reports which were sent to all the main agencies involved in the family's care.

After a few weeks the mother felt sufficiently confident to allow the health visitor and social worker to start visiting again. Within two months the home aide was able to withdraw her support. A home help was then introduced and worked about twenty hours a week in the home.

The health visitor and hospital described the triplets' progress as remarkable. The mother herself seemed to be coping better and with the help of the home aide and home help she started attending a hospital out-patient department for her own problems.

Bristol medical social work project for unsupported parents

The Barclay Report on the role and tasks of social workers (1982) recognises the importance of the personal social services working with the voluntary sector of care. It also recommends that the preventive aspects of the social worker's role should be strengthened. The next project, though small, highlights some important issues in this type of development. It shows how volunteers working closely with a medical social worker can ensure that women considered to be 'at risk' during pregnancy receive support, care and information for their health.

Objectives   In 1979 a senior medical social worker[2] in Bristol set up a six-month pilot project with the objective of reducing the risk of child abuse and neglect in a few families identified to be 'at risk' during pregnancy and at the time of the birth of the babies.

In the course of their normal work, the medical social workers at the Bristol Maternity Hospital have referred to them all expectant mothers from the antenatal clinic who are unmarried, unsupported or who have other social or personal problems. The majority of these mothers receive some support from relatives and friends or other helping agencies. A small minority have no one to whom they can turn for help.

Ideally, many of this latter group should receive some social work in the form of assessment, practical help, emotional support, counselling or liaison with the different agencies who may be involved in their care. At the time of the project the necessary resources for this were not available from the social services department. The senior medical social worker turned, instead, to volunteers.

The volunteers and their work   Four volunteers were recruited with the help of the Bristol Council of Voluntary Service. Three had previously worked in voluntary schemes visiting families. The fourth volunteer was a former social worker. Their ages ranged from thirty-two to forty-five years. All four volunteers were mothers with children of their own.

In the six-month period of the project, two thousand and twenty-one mothers gave birth at the Bristol Maternity Hospital and four hundred and fifty of these were referred to the team of medical social workers. Twenty-nine of these referrals had five or more potential 'risk factors' on a list of fourteen such factors. Each of these had been chosen to indicate possible difficulties in coping with the new baby: an unwanted pregnancy, a history of emotional deprivation in the mother's own childhood, the separation of mother and baby after birth or abnormal parental reactions to the baby's demands. Seven of these women were allocated a volunteer on the grounds that no other social work agencies were offering support. The families included an immature and severely depressed mother, a prostitute who was living in very poor housing conditions, a 19-year-old and her partner, both with criminal records for violence and an educationally subnormal girl of nineteen who, after the birth of the baby, married an illiterate man who was not the child's father.

The way in which the volunteers worked with their families varied according to the parents' needs. They visited them at least once a week but frequently more often than this. Their main role was to befriend the parents, foster the parent/child relationship and, where appropriate, give mothering to the mother herself. They offered practical help, for instance by baby-sitting and shopping. They also encouraged and assisted the mother to use the relevant services, such as clinics, social services and various types of pre-school daycare.

Role of the medical social worker The contribution of the medical social worker was central to the pilot project's success. She initiated, supervised and co-ordinated it. She selected and trained the volunteers. All the cases in the project remained on her own case load and were therefore her responsibility. She saw every volunteer individually for at least an hour every month for advice and counselling. The social worker also had to be available to volunteers both in and out of normal working hours, as they were expected to telephone her whenever they had problems. As a group, they met with her on five occasions during the six-month period.

All this work was done voluntarily by the medical social worker, in addition to her normal and busy workload. She emphasised that if the project had continued her role should have been taken over by a paid and full-time project co-ordinator/supervisor with the appropriate training.

End of the project At the end of the project, three of the families were taken on by social workers in the local authority social services department and two were accepted by a voluntary social work agency. One family maintained a close involvement with a health visitor. The volunteer attached to the remaining family continued to visit them on a friendly basis after the project ended.

Although there has been no formal evaluation of this project, the medical social worker sought the views of the medical and social work staff involved in the project. These were favourable. They had been reassured by the careful selection, training and support of the volunteers who were experienced in visiting and working with families, and they recognised that extra support had been given to some of the most needy families who would not otherwise have been helped. The volunteers' work seemed to have lessened the day-to-day levels of stress in these parents' lives. This in itself may have resulted in healthier pregnancies and a reduction in illness in the babies' early months of life. In several instances the volunteers succeeded in getting health care to the families when they would probably not have received it otherwise.

Funding   Apart from goodwill, the whole of the project ran on a grant of £95 from the social services department. This was given to cover the volunteers' expenses. To continue the scheme would have cost more — the money for a full-time co-ordinator's salary, the office and administrative costs and the volunteers' expenses. But it could be argued that such relatively small investments in this type of social care scheme might result in long-term savings for the health and social services. For instance, a reduction in medical complications in these high-risk pregnancies could save costly inpatient obstetric and neonatal care. A decrease in the incidence of family breakdown could reduce the need for expensive residential care from social services. This seems the type of project which should be considered for Joint Finance (see page 83).

Neighbourhood-based social service teams

The last development to be discussed here moves the initiative for prevention from small, often 'once-off' schemes, to the organisation and management of whole social services departments.

The Barclay Report (1982) on the role and tasks of social workers (National Institute for Social Work 1982) suggests that the philosophy of prevention and community involvement should be central to the way in which social services departments are organised. The recommendations of the report, if acted upon, may result in an increase in the availability of resources for preventive health care, in its widest sense.

> The working party believes that if social needs of citizens are to be met in the last years of the twentieth century, the personal social services must develop a close working partnership with citizens, focussing more closely on the community and its strengths. A move towards what we are calling community social work is the start of such a development.
>
> (*Ibid.* para. 13.1)

Community social work depends upon an attitude of mind in all social workers from the director of the department or agency to front line workers which regards members of the public as partners in the provision of social care.   (*Ibid.* para. 13.2)

There may be many different ways of developing this community approach in social work. Some are already well tried — for instance the attachment of social workers to health centres. Others include the decentralisation of whole area teams so that social services staff are based in small neighbourhood units. As the aim of some of these newer types of development is to work closely with primary health care teams, I will describe their key features.

Most of these neighbourhood- (or 'patch'-) based social services teams have developed independently of each other — yet they share certain common characteristics (Hadley, R. and McGrath, M. 1980). The fieldworkers concentrate their efforts on communities of about five to seven thousand who usually live in a circum- scribed geographical area. They reorientate their work towards prevention, acknowledging the community itself as the major provider of care and an important resource in dealing with problems referred to the social services team. It is this latter characteristic which marks out the community orientated type of social work as a significant departure from current social work practice. A recurring theme in the description of neighbourhood- based social services is the development of close links with all local services, such as general practitioners, health visitors, district nurses, schools and the police, as well as the promotion and co-ordination of work through neighbours, friends and volunteers.

It is important that this new type of social services area team organisation is evaluated and examined in more detail. At the time of writing, this is being done in at least two schemes — Normanton, Wakefield,[3] and Dinnington, South Yorkshire.[4] In Normanton, a DHSS-funded research project is evaluating the way in which the area team has worked since it was divided into three 'patch' teams in 1976. Among many other factors being examined are the changes in health service liaison produced by this reorganisation.

Dinnington patch scheme   The Dinnington patch scheme, a five- year project funded by urban aid, is based in a South Yorkshire mining village that is experiencing rising levels of unemployment. There is a well defined population of approximately seven thousand people. One general practice of eight doctors covers almost all the village, while a health visitor and the district nurses work from a nearby health clinic. Staff of the housing and education welfare departments are also based in offices in the village. Previously, social services were administered from Maltby, a town five miles away.

The results of a small pilot study in 1978 showed that the relationships between the statutory local and health authority services were often haphazard, being left mainly to the individual efforts of those involved, without any systematic encouragement from their managements. Links between local voluntary groups and statutory services were minimal. After discussion between the local and health authorities, it was decided to create a village-centred inter-departmental team to consist of two social workers and a housing assistant. They are based in an office near the centre of the village and only a short distance from the GPs' surgery and the health clinic. The Assistant Home Help Organiser for the area also works from this office. It is hoped that the close proximity of workers from different services will improve working relationships, especially between the health and social services.

The major objectives of the team's work have been defined as:

— to increase the resources available to meet the community's needs by promoting and supporting voluntary and informal care through the statutory services
— to meet 'consumer' needs better; to meet the needs of more people at the same unit cost as the existing services
— to enable people to ask for help earlier; to identify people who need help earlier; to therefore reduce the number of 'crisis' referrals.

A three-year evaluation study of the scheme, funded by the DHSS, commenced in 1980. It includes a series of research projects examining the processes and problems involved in setting up such a scheme, and also studies the project teams' interactions with the health professionals in the village. This research is now well under way. (For further descriptions of this project readers are referred to Bayley, M. *et al.* 1981.)

Although this type of neighbourhood-based organisation may be advantageous in some areas, it is important to emphasise that it is not favoured universally (see for instance the minority report — appendix B — of the Barclay Committee Report 1982). It runs counter to the trend of increasing professionalisation and special-isation in many social services departments. It appears, however, that the number of social services teams who have reorganised their work on a patch basis has increased in recent years.

In conclusion

The schemes described in this chapter indicate how the resources and skills of the personal social services can play an important role in promoting health in pregnancy and early childhood. They can improve economic, environmental and behavioural factors which might otherwise adversely affect people's health and development. This is particularly important at a time when the incidence of family poverty appears to be increasing. They can also assist the families with whom they work to acquire the health care they need. By the nature of referrals to social service departments, these parents and children may often have an above average risk of ill-health.

It seems important that ways are found to encourage greater collaboration in areas of shared interest between social service departments and health authorities and the family practitioner services. The government should consider urgently ways of promoting the use of Joint Finance (from health authority budgets) by local authorities. It should be used imaginatively to develop further collaborative health and social service schemes to promote the health of families, particularly those who are most at risk because of their impoverished material environments. The training of social workers and health professionals should reflect their overlapping areas of interest in preventive health care in pregnancy and early childhood.

Notes

1 County Home Care Organiser, Social Services Department, PO Box 30, Avon House North, Bristol BS99 7NB.
2 Rosemary Ineichen, Principal Medical Social Worker, Southmead Hospital, Bristol BS10 5NB.
3 SCAN, 10 Talbot Street, Normanton, Wakefield, W. Yorkshire.
4 Dr M. Bayley, Department of Sociological Studies, University of Sheffield, Sheffield S10 2TN.

8 Health and the voluntary sector

> 'Some of our present statutory services originated from causes taken up by voluntary organisations . . . Voluntary effort remains at the heart of such services and at local, regional and national levels is often directed towards innovative work and work at the boundaries of existing services. It can complement, enhance and extend the statutory contribution. It can bring a dimension of commitment, diversity and experiment which improves the quality of life and encourages individual self-confidence. But voluntary organisations need support and help in their work . . .'   (DHSS 1981a para 3.1)

In my search for ways of increasing the availability of preventive health care to families in pregnancy and early childhood, I have been struck by the number of projects that arise in the voluntary sector of care.[1]   They range from small, informal networks of family support provided by unpaid neighbours, to mutual-aid groups, and include nationwide schemes mounted by large voluntary organisations involving paid and professionally trained staff.   The relationships of these different schemes to the health and other statutory services vary from relatively independent groups to those whose work falls under the direction of the service professionals (see chapter 7 page 88). This chapter is concerned with the work of the former more independent schemes.

The government is attempting to expand the role of the voluntary sector in the health and social services in a variety of ways that includes schemes to facilitate voluntary work by the unemployed (DHSS 1981b). The discussion which follows centres on reasons for welcoming this expansion. Some mention of the limitations of the voluntary sector must, however, be made, and to omit the caution and fears which have been expressed during this study by volunteers and health workers alike would be wrong.

— Anxiety is expressed about the consequences of expanding volunteering when there is low pay within certain parts of the health service and rising levels of unemployment outside it. It will be tragic if the special contribution which the voluntary sector can make to health care is endangered by the political wrangle which these policies may create between governments, workers and trade unions.

— Fears are raised that voluntary organisations may be swamped with the sudden influx of volunteers which could result from the new schemes for unemployed people. This might threaten the efficiency and effectiveness of their existing work.

— Adequate investment should be made in paid and trained staff to select, prepare, monitor and support the new volunteers; also to find and match them with suitable work (The Volunteer Centre 1982). This needs a certain amount of secure long-term funding. A recent survey of social services departments shows that owing to the financial constraints placed on them, 65 per cent have had to cut their grants to voluntary bodies (BASW Social Context Advisory Panel 1981). This may undermine the viability of the voluntary sector at source.

— Limitations exist in the availability of volunteers for the families and neighbourhoods that need them most (Hatch, S. 1981). Voluntary work tends, largely, to be a middle-class preserve (OPCS 1983c). Research has shown that the fashionable notion of poor people somehow banding together to help themselves may often be quite unreal (Knight, B. and Hayes, R. 1981).

— Traditionally, voluntary work with children and other dependent people has relied heavily on women. However, the changing role and pattern of employment of women may now affect their availability for this type of care.

— Health professionals do not always appreciate what volunteers can do. This may lead to the misuse or neglect of their skills and experience.

— There seems a danger that certain characteristics of the voluntary sector's ways of working may be thought to be peculiar to them. Some probably are: their ability to offer mutual aid and a befriending rather than a professional relationship. But flexibility and innovatory ways of working, often noted as the hallmarks of voluntary schemes, are characteristics which should be encouraged within the statutory services, too. Because of the resource implications, it is unreasonable to leave the research and development of new ways of delivery care primarily to the voluntary sector. Its main base should be within the statutory services.

The wellbeing of the voluntary sector's development in preventive health care may depend on these issues being given adequate attention. But meanwhile there is little doubt that this sector of care has a very particular contribution to make (see for instance Allen, R. and Purkis, A. 1983). In this chapter I will illustrate some of the voluntary sectors' ways of working which may enable them to contact families whom the health services find difficult to reach. Four characteristics have recurred frequently in the projects I have studied. They often seem to differentiate the voluntary from the professional approach to providing care by:

— offering support through non-professional befriending relationships
— gaining acceptance by sharing experiences common to the volunteers and parents
— becoming specialists in identifying and meeting the needs of minority groups
— making contact with large numbers of families through innovatory schemes using the television and radio, linked to 'phone-in services.

Unfortunately, it is impossible to mention all the schemes which illustrate these characteristics; therefore, I will describe in detail a few of the most outstanding examples.

Support through friendship

The families who most need to convey their health problems to professionals, and receive care and information which they can understand, are often those who have the least education, income and social status. The distance between their worlds and the professionals' can be enormous.

The work of many voluntary schemes suggest that volunteers can sometimes bridge these social gaps with a befriending, rather than a professional relationship (see, for instance, Humphries, B. 1976). By visiting and supporting families in their homes, the volunteers can gradually help parents to gain confidence in their own abilities and in their contacts with the statutory services. The story of a single parent with five children (three already in care), whose 6-week-old baby was being fed on custard, potato and milk, illustrates this.

> Not surprisingly the baby was being constantly sick and was losing weight. The health visitor ("What does she know, she'd never even had children herself") and the social worker ("she'll only take the other two off me") had great difficulty in gaining access to the home. At the request of these workers, a mother, who herself had been visited by a volunteer when she had been a single parent with five children, was introduced to the family. Understanding the mother's fear of professionals (two of her own children had been taken into care many years earlier) she was immediately accepted as a friend and was able to gain the mother's confidence and offer her practical advice and help. Throughout her work this volunteer kept in close touch with

the family's health visitor and social worker. Six months later the health visitor reported that the mother had started attending the child health clinic regularly and welcomed her when she visited her at home. The baby was growing and developing well.

(A Home-Start family, Leicester)

Home-Start, Leicester

The work of Home-Start[2] shows the important role which volunteers can play in preventive health care by offering families support and care through friendship. This project has been the subject of a four-year evaluation study, sponsored by the SSRC, from which a part of the data that follows is taken (Van der Eyken 1982).

Finance and volunteers' expenses Home-Start, Leicester, began in 1973 with an urban aid grant, which was augmented later by funds from the Inner Area Programme. In 1982 the scheme's total funding for the year amounted to £40,000, which covered the salaries of three full-time organisers and one full-time secretary, plus the cost of office accommodation, telephone, postage, stationery and training courses. The repayment of the expenses of the 100 or so volunteers amounted to £5,922. This sum reflects Home-Start's philosophy that volunteering should not cost the volunteers any of their own money. Volunteers' expenses cover day-to-day items, like travel and telephoning, and sometimes include costs of cleaning, replacing or repairing anything of their own which might be damaged in the course of their work.

Relation with the statutory services To return to the scheme's early days. Before the first Home-Start volunteers were recruited or the first family visited, a professional support group of senior representatives from the health authority, the social services and education departments of the local authority, the DHSS, the Leicester Council for Voluntary Service and the local Voluntary Worker's Bureau was established. The first organiser of Home-Start, who initiated the project, described this group as vital both in establishing credibility with the departments and agencies which each of its members represented and in ongoing support.

The organiser recalled the development of her relationship with the health services — a story repeated in almost identical phrases by several other voluntary initiatives. It seems that the process of establishing trust is, by its nature, a long and gradual one.

The health services gave us a tough time at the beginning, not least because we proposed calling our volunteers 'home visitors', which abbreviated to HVs, the same as the health visitors! I was invited to address our branch of the Royal College of

Nursing, and was almost literally shredded. However, they did
send me a bouquet of flowers the next day, and shortly after-
wards the first few referrals from health visitors were received.
Now, miraculously, health visitors are our staunchest allies . . .
I am sure they were justifiably worried at first that these
unqualified women were coming in to take over their jobs.
Now we work very successfully side by side.

The volunteers   The majority of volunteers are recruited through
the local Voluntary Workers' Bureau. The only qualification is
that the applicant should be a parent. Of the ninety-four volunteers recruited between 1974 and 1978, just over a third had only
their natural qualification of 'parent'. All but two were women
and the average age was thirty-seven, in a range between twenty-
two to sixty-four years. Just under half the volunteers recruited
in 1974 and 1975 were still working with Home-Start in August
1978 (Van der Eyken 1982). The considerable length of service
probably owes much to the careful attention given to the volunteer's compulsory course of preparation and to continued training
and support.

All Home-Start volunteers must attend a preliminary course
which helps them to decide if they are suited to the work and can
give the necessary commitment of time and energy. The course
usually lasts for a full day every week for ten weeks. Evening or
weekend courses are occasionally arranged. Basic information is
given about child development, welfare rights, the ethics of visiting
other people in their homes, the range of services available to
families and the roles of the various professionals involved in
them.

The volunteers learn about non-accidental injuries to children;
a health visitor talks about her profession and explains the importance of immunising children and checking their hearing, vision
and general development regularly. She discusses how the volunteers can encourage the families they visit to use these preventive
health services. The volunteers visit day nurseries, nursery classes
and playgroups, and go on joint visits to families with experienced
volunteers.

Providing adequate support for each volunteer is considered a
top priority by the Home-Start organisers[3] as the volunteers could
easily be swamped by the types of problem they were dealing with
and by the depth of their own involvement. The organisers are in
regular contact with each volunteer by telephone or meetings.
Volunteers are also encouraged to form mutual self-help support
groups with three or four in a group. Refresher courses, occasional
lectures, discussions, informal coffee evenings and lunches are also
held regularly. In all their work volunteers are encouraged to seek

advice, when necessary, from the professionals who work with 'their' families.

Referrals   Home-Start operates an 'open door' policy for referrals, accepting all cases.   Many of them have complex and sometimes apparently intractable social and family problems.   Indeed, an analysis of the referred cases in the four-year period up to April 1978 showed that a sixth of them were either on the 'at risk register', were on supervision orders or were said by the referee to be likely candidates for institutional care (Van der Eyken 1982). In 1978 it was estimated that 90 per cent of the families were from the inner city areas of Leicester, 40 per cent were single parents and 11 per cent were immigrants.

About a third of Home-Start's referrals come from health visitors, a third from social workers and a further 10 per cent or so are self-referrals.   The rest tend to come from agencies such as child guidance clinics, the probation service, infant schools and family service units (Harrison, M. 1979).   Once referred to Home-Start, each family is visited by one of the organisers to assess their particular needs and the type of volunteer who could best meet them.

The success of matching appropriate Home-Start volunteers to the families referred is crucial to the success of the scheme. Between March 1974 and March 1978 Home-Start found a suitable volunteer for three-quarters of their referrals.   During this time only five relationships between the allocated volunteers and the families broke down, when the visitor was replaced with another (Van der Eyken, 1982).

Writing about the matching process, the organiser who set up Home-Start admitted that it is mainly intuitive, based on close knowledge of the volunteers, their abilities, interests and backgrounds, and those of the families referred.

Home visits   Each volunteer usually visits two or three families. In August 1982 just over 100 volunteers were visiting about 200 families in Leicester.   A survey of volunteers showed that on average they spent six hours a week with their families in addition to keeping notes, attending meetings and contacting the organiser and other fieldworkers involved in their cases (Van der Eyken, 1982).   On this basis and with the grant of £40,000 in 1982, Home-Start's volunteers were providing the equivalent number of hours of about fifteen full-time workers.

The volunteers' work with their families varies according to the families' needs and the volunteers' abilities.   Volunteers try to offer a friendship that is consistently caring and non-judgemental. They can give practical help by looking after the children, clearing and cleaning up the home or doing the shopping; again, they may play an educational role with the parents and children. They give emotional support by listening to parents' worries and anxieties. Some volunteers restrict themselves to their regular home visiting, while others include the families in their own lives, taking them on outings and involving them with their friends.

Collaboration with all the statutory services is an important part of Home-Start's work. Whenever a volunteer is introduced to a new family, the referring agent and the family's health visitor is informed of her name, address and telephone number, and she is given similar details of other workers involved with the family to whom she may turn for advice or support.

The organiser of Home-Start gave many instances of the volunteers' success in reaching families who need intensive support for their health and development. The following are extracts from her notes. The main identifying features of families have been altered to preserve their anonymity:

— Three young children had been in care because they were left alone in the house while parents went out at night. Mother pregnant. HSV did babysitting at first, then gradually accepted by family as a friend, who could support all of them during the day too. Very close liaison with health visitor, midwife and doctor.

— 18-year-old single mother brought up in care herself, expecting third baby. Second child died (cot death) a year ago, aged 15 weeks. Mother finds it virtually impossible to make and then keep friends. No one constant in her life. HSV requested to befriend her during pregnancy, so a relationship would be established and she could begin intensive support once the baby was born. This she did, despite several attempts at rejection by the mother. Not an ideal situation even now, but the child is 15 months old, developing well, and at least the mother 'has a family of my own'.

— Agoraphobic mother with toddler daughter. HSV took own children to visit and extend her world. Also helped with visits to clinic and supported mother through subsequent pregnancy.

— Mother with epilepsy and history of frequent hospitalisation and ill-health. Husband at work. Neighbours 'didn't want to know'. HSV introduced. First 'friend' the mother had had. Gained confidence through this, and developed interest in herself and her children through the visits. Got to know the neighbours, who began to be involved. HSV able to withdraw.

Spreading the scheme beyond Leicester   By the summer of 1982 there were twenty-two other schemes of this type operating in

England, with a further twenty well on the way to being funded. A Home-Start consultancy service was established in 1981 to assist in their development and to help in initiating more. The staff consists of two experienced Home-Start workers, one full- and one part-time, who are funded by the London Law Trust. An additional grant from the DHSS allowed the team to include an Information and Development Officer and a part-time secretary.

In summary, the work of Home-Start illustrates the potential of this type of voluntary scheme for preventive family health care. It shows how meticulous attention to organisation, recruiting, preparation, matching and support of volunteers has led to a service which can complement that provided by the statutory services. There is a special role for volunteers who can approach families without the burden of professional status and all that it implies. They are able to give families a type of caring support which, by the nature of things, can rarely be provided by the professionals in the health and social services.

The relevance of parents' own experience

Within two months of Claire's birth, we needed help when we were told at the hospital that she had a heart murmur. Immediately I got home, I rang Mrs C. and talked for a very long time . . . Within an hour, I had two telephone calls from parents in the group whose children had heart murmurs.

(A mother writing about a mutual-aid scheme,
Southend-on-Sea, Essex)

The above extract illustrates the special ability of mutual-aid groups to reach parents at times of stress. Volunteers who have experienced a particular situation can offer unique understanding and knowledge, which can sometimes give them necessary acceptability when parents withdraw from other sources of help through their grief, depression, guilt or sheer exhaustion.

Many mutual-aid groups have been contacted for this study — twins clubs,[4] stillbirth groups,[5] groups for parents who feel violent towards their children[6] and groups for specific types of childhood illness and disability.[7] Their histories tend to confirm the findings of the Wolfenden Committee (1978) that mutual-aid organisations specialising in health-related problems are increasing. Some are locally based; others are part of regional or even national organisations.

The potential of this expanding community resource of organised mutual aid should not be underestimated in health care. The following accounts of three different mutual-aid groups illustrate ways in which voluntary organisations like these attempt to reach parents with special health needs.

Stillbirth mutual-aid groups

With approximately seven stillbirths in every thousand deliveries, stillbirth (see chap. 1 note 1) remains a common tragedy (OPCS 1982b). In 1976, *The Guardian* carried an article in which a journalist vividly described her own experience of a stillbirth. She highlighted the unique problems of parents mourning the loss of a baby which lacks a living identity (*Lancet* 1977); and of the gap in many professionals' knowledge about these parents' special needs. Doctors, nurses and midwives on the antenatal and postnatal wards often found it difficult to readjust their caring for those facing death rather than birth.

The article occasioned correspondence, which included the suggestion that parents of a stillborn baby might find help from others who had undergone the experience of stillbirth. A psychiatric social worker, who was the mother of a stillborn child, took on this task voluntarily. In a letter published in the national press she appealed to mothers to tell her what information they lacked at the time of their stillbirths. She received nearly 200 replies, many of which recounted feelings of depression and guilt that sometimes persisted for years, and the failure of hospital staff to recognise the special needs of the bereaved.

Within two years a booklet was produced for parents of stillbirth, perinatal and neonatal deaths. A group of interested doctors, together with the Health Education Council and MIND, helped with preparation and publication. Entitled 'The Loss of Your Baby',[8] it has been widely advertised and distributed through the health service.

Between 1977 and 1978, several mothers who had experienced stillbirths formed a central organisation to disseminate advice. This was later known as the Stillbirth and Perinatal Death Association. The two main aims of the association are to form a national network of support for mothers of stillbirths, perinatal and neonatal deaths, while also preparing teaching material to inform doctors, nurses and midwives of the particular problems which these parents face. As this association has become known, referrals have been received from a wide range of sources — the press, voluntary organisations and doctors, midwives and health visitors.

Through the central association, bereaved mothers can contact others who have had similar experiences and live in the local area. In 1977 only one local stillbirth group was known to exist. By 1980 the number had increased to just over fifty, spread over England, Scotland and Wales. One of the originators of the association commented:

Clearly the way we had to operate at the beginning was far from ideal — we often wondered who we were putting in touch with whom and what complications might arise. But it was all very well for the professionals to tell us to move slowly and in the 'proper way' — you couldn't tell women they had to wait for years until the professionals changed and the services recognised their needs. Their pain was now, and it had to be met.

The association stresses the importance of training for their new 'befriending' parents. A leaflet has been prepared to advise how to make initial contact with a bereaved parent and how to cope with some of the problems they may find when visiting. In a few areas professionals such as psychologists and psychiatrists offer counselling training courses for members of the local stillbirth groups.

Gradually, midwives, health visitors and GPs are recognising the useful role which these experienced volunteers may play in the management of parents' grief after a stillbirth. Where trust and a working relationship has been established these health professionals may be key publicity points for the work of local groups.

In some hospitals the obstetrician or ward sister gives newly bereaved parents a card with the address and telephone number of the local stillbirth group, together with the booklet 'The Loss of Your Baby'. Unfortunately this method of contact is seldom successful, as parents are usually too depressed to respond. More successful is the personal explanation, offered by the midwife or doctor, of the help which members of a stillbirth group can give. If the parents feel they would like to talk to another parent and agree to their name and address being passed on, the member of staff then contacts the local group organiser. She, in turn, arranges for the newly bereaved parents to be visited before they leave hospital or soon after their return home.

The nature and objectives of these home visits are described in the association's leaflet 'Notes on Initial Visit by a Befriending Parent'.

You too have lost a baby — that is an immediate reason for trust and sympathy between you and they know that you understand personally something of the terrible blow they have received, and their pain . . . Make clear who you are and why you are there, and try to share her feelings. Do not reassure her too quickly; do not get into arguments about her doctor or her care or how she should feel. Listen carefully and respond to how she feels. Remember that each person will react in her own way . . . Accept the way the parents feel and your own limitations — you are befriending, not curing or counselling.

Wherever possible the volunteer gives the parents her 'phone number and encourages them to use it whenever they need to talk about the loss. New parents are also invited to join the local stillbirth group and to attend their regular meetings, where they may gain support from other members.

Perhaps more than most volunteering, visiting bereaved parents demands much attention to the volunteer's own needs. Wherever possible, support is given by the group organiser and by other group members, informally and in group meetings and sometimes by psychologists and doctors.

Mutual-aid groups for parents under stress

The term 'child abuse' refers to situations ranging from the neglect of children's physical and emotional needs to actual violence. The true prevalence of the different types of child abuse is unknown. A figure for England of some 5,000 children affected by violent abuse every year has been suggested (House of Commons Select Committee on Violence in the Family, 1977).

The Select Committee on Violence in the Family considered ways of preventing child abuse. Among others, they recommended that if parents needed advice urgently they should have easy access to a suitable contact (para 63). They further recommended that parents should be encouraged to form mutual-aid groups to help with the stress of raising children and that these groups should consider providing a regular telephone service for parents (para 70).

The history of mutual-aid groups for parents under stress (sometimes known as Parents Anonymous or PA groups) illustrates a voluntary response to provide this type of service. It is important, though, that this development is not seen as a criticism of existing professional services. To quote an organiser of a local group:

> It is a response to a need which individuals have experienced and which they see as impossible for social workers, health visitors or GPs etc. to meet. Indeed we would argue that self-help is a vital part of the helping process and that a professional cannot do what a volunteer parent can.

Influenced by the earlier developments of the American and Canadian Parents Anonymous movement, the first groups in this country were set up in 1975 in Northwood, Nottingham and Brighton. By 1981 some fifty local groups had been established throughout the country, with another ten in preparation. It was not until 1979, when many local groups were already formed, that a central and national organisation was established: Organisations for Parents Under Stress (OPUS). A national co-ordinating committee of OPUS has been formed to help establish new groups, to disseminate information between the groups, to advise on training and to monitor new developments in this type of mutual aid. The national committee is funded by the DHSS and is advised by a panel of experts on parental stress and child abuse. Many professionals also support their local groups by being available to advise volunteers on cases.

Most OPUS groups offer a telephone support service for parents to use at any time. Some also provide befriending home visiting services, drop-in centres and support through group work. It is hoped that the anonymity offered to 'phone callers, together with the rigorous confidentiality of the groups' work, may encourage parents to 'phone when they are too frightened or embarrassed to disclose their identity to the statutory services. It may be at such times that they and their children are most in need of help.

Trained volunteer parents, many having experienced extreme stress when raising their own children, answer the telephones. They are prepared to listen and to be sympathetic and supportive. The volunteers always try to get the callers to make their own referrals. Frightened parents can sometimes be persuaded to ask for help if they talk with a volunteer who has had to approach professionals in a similar situation. If a child is thought to be in immediate danger, most groups consult with their professional advisers and by-pass the self-referral route. However, Parents Anonymous Croydon and Tanbridge (PACT) reported that in a period of approximately two years and some 1,000 'phone calls, many involving potentially dangerous cases, they had always succeeded in persuading parents to make their own contact with professional help (Ashley, A. 1980).

Before volunteers work with a group they usually have to attend a course of preparation, which varies from group to group according to the type of services provided. The course often includes talks by professionals on their roles in the care of families and the services that are provided. Volunteers are helped also to develop an awareness of the wide range of styles of parenting. Through role-play and discussion they learn how to handle 'phone calls when parents ask for help with violence or neglect to their children. Most groups also insist on regular in-service training for all their volunteers. The national co-ordinating committee has prepared a series of pamphlets[9] to assist groups in these various training schemes.

The number of calls which groups receive appears to be directly related to their success in obtaining publicity. The story of those who manage to achieve radio or television publicity is always the same. Within a few seconds their telephone lines are blocked with queues of anxious parents wanting to talk to someone. If groups do not plan in advance for this enormous response, they may be overwhelmed.

Unfortunately, few OPUS groups have much access to this form of publicity. Most report that a major part of their expenses go towards printing materials for posters and notices to be displayed in clinics, libraries and schools. In some districts health visitors and GPs give parents printed cards describing the groups' work and the address and 'phone number of a contact.

The success of these types of telephone 'help' lines is hard to gauge. It is impossible to know how many potential or actual situations of child abuse exist in the local community and what proportion of these are reached by mutual-aid schemes, rather than by the statutory health and social services.

An analysis of the records of PA Nottingham's 'phone cases between 1976 and 1979 shows that half were thought to have reached a crisis point where help was needed urgently. In 1979, Parents Anonymous Croydon and Tanbridge (PACT) received 306 first-time telephone contacts. From these, they identified 5 cases which involved actual child abuse, 11 cases where child abuse was thought to have been likely and 35 where the volunteers felt that child abuse was possible if circumstances provoked more tension within the home. Of the first group, all the parents received help from various agencies: social services, the NSPCC and the child psychiatric services. About half the other cases were befriended and visited by volunteers; some of them joined a PACT parent support group and all were advised to seek help from professional agencies.

Southend's early visiting scheme for families of Downs Syndrome babies

Downs Syndrome, known also as mongolism, is one of the commonest forms of mental handicap diagnosed, with an estimated incidence of about 17 cases per 10,000 total births. This incidence increases steeply when the mother is aged 35 years or older (Weatherall, J. 1982). The condition can usually be identified soon after birth, and the diagnosis is confirmed by chromosome tests. Studies have shown the grief and shock which parents experience at this time, and the stress which may result from having a mentally handicapped child in the family (Gath, A. 1978; Hannam, C. 1980).

In 1971 the Southend and District Society for Mentally Handicapped Children[10] set up a mutual-aid support group for parents of Downs children in their first two years of life. It aims to prevent the breakdown of families by offering them support and information. At the start of the scheme, parents rarely joined for a considerable time after the condition was diagnosed, yet most would have liked immediate support. In some instances, the parents did not learn about the group's existence in time; others hesitated to join as they felt unsure about facing strangers and all that the group implied.

The leader of 0-2 support group, herself the mother of a Downs Syndrome child, approached the local paediatrician and together they devised a new referral system. Now, when a Downs Syndrome baby is diagnosed, a health professional explains the nature of the condition to the parents and helps them to cope with the immediate shock. They are asked if they would like to meet a doctor who deals in services for children in the community together with the mother of an older Downs Syndrome child. If the parents agree, the doctor (a senior clinical medical officer) and parent visit them, usually within forty-eight hours of the news being broken. A second visit is made within a few days to answer any further questions. The parents are then invited to join the 0-2 support group. Before visiting the parents, the doctor member of the team usually telephones the family's GP to tell him of the home-visiting service and to ask if they may see the parents. Health visitors are also contacted.

By mid 1981, nearly ten years after the start of the scheme, the home-visiting team had been called to see the parents of 96 Downs Syndrome babies, sometimes only a few hours after their birth. The volunteer member of the team is available to visit at any time of the day or night, weekday, weekend or bank holiday. A deputy is available to cover her absences.

The following account by the mother of a Downs Syndrome baby shows how this type of scheme may succeed in reaching and supporting parents when they are in acute distress.

> My rejection of my baby Claire was total and complete: I just didn't want to know anything about her. After all, she was a cabbage, no use to herself or anybody else . . . I lay and listened to her breathing and hoped she'd stop. But the nightmare was for real, it was happening and I didn't know what to do or where to turn . . .
>
> Within thirty-six hours of Claire's birth, Dr M., and Mrs C. came to see me and my husband. Mrs C. sat at the end of my bed. 'I know how you feel. I have been through this myself.' Immediately my bubble burst, this bright, cheerful woman knew what I was feeling, she had had a mongol boy herself . . . she was not depressed. Dr M. answered all the medical questions we had been worrying about. Mrs C. explained how important it was to take Claire out and get her accepted into society by neighbours and friends alike. To tell people that she was a mongol, but it didn't matter because we were going to cope and she was going to help us. They told us of physiotherapy exercises to improve Claire's muscles . . . we were told about a

group of parents and how it worked and were invited to attend the next meeting in two weeks' time. We kept Dr M. and Mrs C. for three hours and they left saying that they would be back again in ten days' time to answer any further questions that we had thought of in that time. But, if I was at all worried, or anxious, Mrs C. left her telephone number so that I could contact her . . . we felt so different then. Dr M. and Mrs C. came back as promised and answered all our questions. More important — they sat and listened to us talking and understood.

We went to our first group meeting with great trepidation . . . none of them could have gone through what we had, couldn't have suffered the mental anguish that we had . . . Mrs C. welcomed us. She asked the other parents to tell us about their child and how they had felt when it was born. By the time the third couple were speaking, I realised how wrong I was . . . when it came to our turn to tell the group about Claire, all those pent up feelings flooded from us. These people, strangers 'til this evening, were sitting listening to us and understanding. They knew about the guilt I felt, they knew how difficult it was to tell the first person that she was a mongol.

The success soon became known to other paediatricians and health professionals through conferences and by word of mouth. Referrals began to come from people working in the area surrounding Southend, and to cope with this increased demand, new group leaders were found with the necessary experience and knowledge to form early home-visiting teams and run 0-2 parents' support groups. Now that news of the schemes has spread, home-visiting teams and parents' groups have been established in other health authorities, although the exact number of groups in existence is not known (see also Pugh, G. and Russell, R. 1977).

A specialist role for reaching minority groups

The next characteristic of the voluntary sector's way of working to which I want to draw attention is the ability of its members to identify the unmet, and often unrealised, needs of certain minority groups and to become specialists in meeting them. This is evident in the work of the mutual-aid groups just described. It is also a quality which marks out the work of other types of voluntary organisations established specifically to work with relatively small groups of people — for instance, those with a particular disability or disease.

Gypsies and the Save the Children Fund's health work

Gypsies, sometimes called travellers, are an example of a small minority group whose health needs, though great, are rarely met adequately. The health service's increasing awareness of this group's health problems and the improvements which have occurred in their health care in a few areas owes much to the efforts of the voluntary sector (Lawrie, B. 1983). It seems that even this degree of progress would have been hard to achieve without this sector's specialist knowledge, experience and innovations.

Although much of the evidence on gypsies' health is anecdotal, it suggests they have an abnormally high rate of illness and premature death, particularly in early childhood. Reports frequently describe women going into labour without any previous antenatal care, large numbers of childhood accidents and infections, including polio, and very low levels of immunisation (see for instance Sampson, K. and Stockford, D. 1979). This burden of ill-health is probably associated with factors like the dangerous and insanitory conditions of the sites on which many gypsies camp, their poverty and their lack of education and basic health care.

Providing maternity and pre-school health care for this small, scattered and nomadic group is difficult. Their mobility makes them hard to find and presents problems for continuity of care. Gypsies may be frightened and hostile to health workers who visit them, mistaking them for the various officials who often evict them from their illegal camping sites.[11] Contacting them by post is even more difficult. They frequently lack a postal address acceptable to the GPO and can rarely read.

Sadly, it seems that another major obstacle to gypsies' health care is prejudice. Reports indicate that the lack of tolerance which gypsies experience from society in general also occurs within the health service. They tell of hostility to gypsies from fellow patients. GPs and health authorities have sometimes found it difficult to provide them with health care, even when this was requested (Wiltshire Gypsy Council 1978).

The following account tells of attempts to tackle some of these difficult and sensitive issues. It focuses mainly on the work of one volunteer who pioneered the health projects and continues to be a specialist in the field. But this should be seen also in the context of the Save the Children Fund (SCF), a large national voluntary organisation.[12] In 1970, four years after the original volunteer started working on her own with gypsies, she persuaded SCF to take up the problems of gypsy children and their families. A programme was subsequently set up to support her work and to develop other projects throughout the country. In 1982 these involved a total of seventeen paid SCF field staff (including the original worker) and a National Gypsy Liaison Officer based at SCF's London headquarters. Although only the health aspects of SCF's work with gypsies are described here, their other projects include playgroup schemes and schools for gypsy children.

In 1966 a Public Health Inspector, concerned about an un-authorised encampment of six gypsy families in his area in Hert-fordshire, placed an advertisement in the local newspaper.

Help wanted. Urgent social problems. No pay.
No thanks.

His request was quickly taken up by a mother who had trained in social work and had one year's nursing experience. As she began to visit the site, the families' health needs were immediately apparent. There were six women, all of them pregnant, and none receiving any antenatal care. Of the fifty-three children, none were immunised and several had other health problems requiring attention. By talking with the gypsies and listening to their diffi-culties and fears, the volunteer gradually gained their trust and was able to offer help. Within a year they had been given a permanent camp site, the children were in schools, they were registered with GPs and a health visitor was visiting them. As she became known, the volunteer became increasingly involved with other gypsy families in the county, helping to link them up with the various health, educational and social agencies in the areas where they camped.

In 1976 the volunteer moved to Suffolk and found that her services were still in great demand. Few of the gypsies in her new area were registered with GPs or were known to health visitors. Most of the families were frightened of approaching clinics and surgeries for help.

SCF's mobile caravan   This time the volunteer tried a new solution to these problems — a mobile caravan clinic. Money was raised by numerous fund-raising activities and a donation from SCF. Boys from a nearby school converted the caravan to a plan devised by local doctors and health visitors. Equipment came from various sources, including the health authority.

With the agreement of local travellers, the mobile clinic was launched at the 1978 Midsummer Fair at Cambridge. This is an annual gathering of gypsies lasting for ten days. It attracts to one site about 600 caravans with an attached population of between 2,000 and 3,000 travellers. The health authority provided a clinical medical officer and health visitor for six clinic sessions. The volun-teer was based in the clinic for the duration of the Fair. Antenatal care, postnatal care, family planning, immunisation and develop-mental testing services were provided, as well as general health education. Records were kept of all consultations. SCF designed a special health record card, one half of which was given to the traveller to keep, while the other was kept in the mobile clinic.

The travellers' response to the clinic was a reminder that the business of breaking down barriers of mistrust and misinformation is often a slow one.

I had expected that we would be very busy with queues requesting immunisation, weighing of babies and advice, but this did not happen. The travellers are very reticent about discussing personal affairs with new people. We had to approach them rather on the lines of health visiting in the home. Only after general discussion were they ready to come to the caravan. They were very adamant about not having immunisation apart from polio. (Health Visitor's Report)

Altogether some ninety travellers were seen in the course of the clinics. Just over half of these were children. Parents were uncertain of what the clinic could offer and tended to use it more as a casualty department than for its broader preventive function. Travellers found it hard to accept that the clinical medical officers, unlike general practitioners, could not offer treatment or prescriptions.

Despite these problems the experiment was considered sufficiently successful to repeat it the following summer (1979). The same team of health professionals ran the clinic sessions: familiar faces seemed important.

The number of travellers seeking help increased. The health visitor now reported:

We were immediately inundated with children who remembered us from last year and we took this opportunity to test their eyes . . . I felt this year more than last the need to health visit in its actual sense. The occasional times I did speak to the families in their homes, the women were much more communicative.

Development of special health education materials Through this type of work it has become apparent that there is a great need for health education among gypsies. In this respect, the pictures, posters and leaflets available through the NHS health education services are of little use. They can rarely be read and are likely to cause offence if the pictures are at all intimate.

With the help of a senior nursing officer and a local health visitor, the volunteer has prepared a tape/slide set, explaining the various procedures carried out during children's developmental tests. Its style and language have been chosen carefully so that the information will be understood easily by travellers. Another tape/slide set on family planning has been designed so that it is acceptable to this group; a third is now available on the importance of antenatal care, child care and immunisation.[13]

Although there has been no formal evaluation of these health education materials, they are popular with the gypsies and attract large audiences to the mobile caravan. Whenever possible they are shown with a health visitor present so that the travellers have a natural opportunity to ask questions and get to know her in a familiar and friendly setting.

Influencing health service practice   By its example, the SCF clinic suggests alternative ways by which health professionals can reach travellers. Between the caravan's regular visits to roadside families and appointments at gypsy fairs it has been loaned to various health authorities. In Essex it was used by a health visitor on an unofficial site on which about seventy gypsy families lived. The women were uncertain of how to use clinics and surgeries, except in emergencies, and seemed afraid to visit the health centre. Once the health visitor was based outside the centre, in the SCF caravan, she won their trust and was able to see them regularly. Within nine months she had succeeded in encouraging them to the health centre. The caravan was then transferred on short loan to another community project in York, where links were being formed with the health authority.

SCF have also attempted to influence health service practice surveys. Their first, in 1979, requested details of regional health authorities' health service provision for gypsy families (Sampson and Stockford 1979). The report was sent to every area health authority and prompted several enquiries for the loan of the SCF mobile clinic and advice in the design of health services for gypsies. Most recently (1982) SCF carried out a small study of childhood illnesses and premature death in gypsies in the East Anglian health region.

In summary this scheme has underlined the voluntary sector's specialist role in developing new ways of delivering health care to minority groups. Gradually, the skills of voluntary work have uncovered unmet health needs, found ways to meet them and have informed and persuaded health authorities to respond. In other words, the original volunteer and SCF have played the role of a development agency for the NHS. Managers in the NHS should consider how they can support and benefit from the specialist role of the voluntary sector.

There is perhaps one rider to be added: with a few notable exceptions, GPs have not been involved in these various voluntary efforts to provide health services to gypsies. It seems that family practitioner committees may need to consider special arrangements for the primary health care of this group; and, indeed, for others who have no postal address, such as the inner city homeless.

Communicating by television and radio

These provide a route for reaching parents and children by the million, giving immediate access to their everyday lives. However, with the exception of health education officers it seems that many health professionals are reluctant to experiment with these rapidly changing and expanding technologies of communication. This may be due to many factors: professional status and maintaining a certain public image, codes of professional conduct, accountability to large public organisations and lack of appropriate media training.

In contrast, there appears to be an increasing number of voluntary schemes working with TV and radio to contact families, identify their needs and locate and develop new networks of community resources to meet them. Fewer schemes were identified working with TV than with local radio, probably because of high production costs of TV and the size of the population covered by regional TV companies. Their viewers often live far beyond the areas served by local voluntary groups. This situation may change with the introduction of the IBA's Channel Four and the obligation of the new regional companies to employ community and continuing education officers. These innovations are likely to encourage growth in social action and educational broadcasting by television as well as local radio. Much of this will probably involve volunteers in the community,[14] and may be important for preventive health care programmes in the future.

For the time being, however, radio, particularly local radio, seems to be the most accessible broadcasting media for voluntary groups wanting to make contact with a large audience in their local area. The massive expansion of local radio throughout the country that is planned for the next decade is likely to be an important factor in the development of this type of work (IBA 1981; BBC 1983). The two projects which follow indicate ways in which local radio, linked to telephone services, can contribute to preventive health care.

NERDT and the Child Care Switchboard experiment

'He's doing it now. Can you hear him? . . . wait a bit, I'll move the phone so you can hear him properly.'

A terrible thudding mixed with the noise of a sobbing baby comes down the line. The child is banging his head against the wall at home.

'Just stop him doing it, *stop* him', we say.

Maureen picks up the baby. We pose the obvious question. Has she taken Darren to see the doctor?

'Well, I did but it wasn't any good. I'm pregnant again and

he's gone off six months since. The doctor (she's about 28) didn't ask me why I'd come. She just said was I taking, you know, precautions. I said "What bloody business is it of yours. You haven't got any kids, you aren't even bloody married." Bloody cheek. So I walked out and I've not been back for anything from that day to this. And I *won't* go back either. I'm not having that.'   (Jackson, B. 1982)

The National Educational Research and Development Trust (NERDT) is a voluntary organisation developing ways of meeting the education and social needs of children and their families. In 1977, with the help of the BBC, the organisation's late director, Brian Jackson, pioneered a Child Care Switchboard experiment with a budget of less than £6,000. Its aim is to link parents with problems to sources of help by means of local radio and telephone. Much of the information in the following description has been taken from the report of the project (Jackson, B. 1982).

The Child Care Switchboard[15] was given a total of twenty-four hours live broadcasting spread between six local BBC radio stations in England. The Switchboard's length of operation in any one centre lasted from between three and seven days, and included news items, interviews, 'phone-ins, magazine programmes and outside broadcasts from streets, schools and factories. Health visitors and doctors were among the many professionals involved.

Preparation and publicity   From the start, a research worker/co-ordinator was employed to go from centre to centre finding out the necessary information about the local resources and services to which families could be referred. Meetings were held with senior managers from health authorities and education and social services departments to explain the aims of the project and seek their co-operation. Voluntary organisations were also approached for their help.

In each centre a 'phone number was widely advertised for parents with problems to call.

You couldn't get near Nottingham Castle on the day the Switchboard opened without glimpsing shoppers wearing the special Switchboard badge. We tried to persuade the BBC to come out of their studio and invite callers from housing estates, shopping precincts, schools and factories. We littered the pubs with colourful beer mats inviting a 'phone call so that an anxious father worried about his child might just put 2p in that coin box.

Callers and their problems   People were offered the choice of remaining completely anonymous and talking over a private line or of sharing their problems with listeners over the 'phone-link which was broadcast 'live'. Although the public line was limited to the broadcasting time allocated to the Switchboard, the private line remained open for much longer.

Each radio station kept a log book of number of calls received, presenting problems and, if given, names and addresses of the callers. During the 127 hours of access, over all the public and private telephone lines, 508 people rang and discussed a child-related problem. However, the actual demand was probably many times greater as lines became blocked.

The average length of the calls was twenty minutes; many were considerably longer. About half the callers agreed to discuss their worries over the public line (heard over the air) with the other half speaking on the private lines. Over the air, about 40 per cent of callers remained anonymous, in contrast to those on the private lines who nearly all gave names and addresses, thus allowing the project to reach them with help. The project had expected the majority of enquiries to concern pre-school children, but found in practice that no particular age group presented more frequently than another. Seventy per cent of the calls came from mothers, 20 per cent from fathers and the remainder from grandparents, aunts, uncles, neighbours, friends or older children.

Many problems were similar to those encountered regularly by GPs, health visitors, teachers and others working with young children. Calls concerned behaviour difficulties, bedwetting, speech, hearing, and vision problems, physical handicaps, stresses of the single parent and despair after a child's death. Some callers identified children seriously at risk of physical and emotional abuse.

Despite the gravity of some problems it was notable that many callers said they had never received help from the statutory or voluntary agencies. To quote from the project report — 'They were surrounded by services to which they seemed to have no means of access.' Extracts from the telephone calls illustrated this.

I rang my doctor and there was an ansaphone on. That was no good to me, so I rang you.

There's a little girl over the road, about four, moved here with her parents about two years ago but she never comes out. We only get glimpses — she's never seen daylight. The curtains are drawn, no windows ever opened, it's so senseless . . . Does she have to die before anyone will do anything?

Project's degree of success   Twenty callers were visited three months after the project ended. It was apparent that even in this small sample of predominantly working-class families, many had received assistance as a result of their contact with the Switchboard.

> After I rang the Child Care Switchboard up, they came to us
> like flies round a jampot. Until then we'd had nothing.
> (Mother of a partially blind boy with Marfans Syndrome)

The follow-up study suggested too that through radio, perhaps a few severely depressed and anxious parents could be encouraged to make a 'phone call for help — something which they might otherwise find difficult.

> That Child Care week on Radio Nottingham was sent from
> heaven to me. I can't describe what I was like. I wanted to
> murder Lee. I know it's wrong, I know it's silly and after all
> she's only three — and I love her. But I had this feeling, this
> feeling to hit her and kill her all the time. I locked myself in
> the lavatory. And I just lay there on the floor by the pan crying
> and crying . . . But I wasn't locking her *out*, I was locking
> myself in . . . but that morning when the Children's Care broad-
> casts were on — I knew they were going to be on, I'd heard
> them say so, so I was listening. That morning I sat listening to
> them and I thought Oh God, I wish someone would come and
> talk to me. I knew I couldn't do it over the air, I'd have gone to
> pieces. Then I listened every morning, hoping someone like me
> would come on with a similar problem. Until I heard the
> Switchboard the feeling was that bad in my mind I didn't know
> what to ask. And then I said to myself, get on the 'phone and
> ask, ring while there's a chance. So I went out and the 'phone
> was vandalised. And the next one was too. I had to go to the
> shops by the roundabout a mile or so and then found one that
> worked. Well they sent a social worker especially to me and she
> said I'd got to go into hospital for a week. The nurses and the
> doctor were very good to me . . .

The Child Care Switchboard experiment was only intended to test briefly ways in which local radio can reach families with problems. Within its short time-span it proved sufficiently successful with radio producers and the public to suggest that this idea should be developed further and on a more permanent basis.

> We have hit a vein of need and opportunity: there are lots of
> people who need help and want help, but don't know how to
> get it. And there is also a radio opportunity. What *better* way
> is there of reaching large numbers of people than local radio,
> when the need is two-way? It is not just broadcasting at people
> but involving their participation . . . a vital part of the Switch-
> board process. More broadcasting of this kind should be done.
> (Extract from Radio Leeds' Station Manager's Report to
> Broadcasting House)

NCH's Family Care Line, Manchester

A project in Manchester has built the experience of the Child Care
Switchboard into a long-term project. Family Care Line[16] is a
radio/phone-in project run jointly by Family Network (a regional
family support service of the National Children's Home) and
Picadilly Radio (Manchester's commercial radio station). It broadcasts twelve thirty-second 'trails' every day, inviting anyone with a
family problem to 'phone the private number to discuss it in
confidence. In addition, Picadilly Radio puts out a half-hour
feature programme every week on different family topics, which
also advertises the service. The 'phone lines are open every weekday from 11.00 am to 3.00 pm and from 7.00 pm to 9.30 pm. An
ansaphone covers the times when the lines are closed, inviting
callers to phone the Samaritans if they need help there and then.

The staff and the radio station　Trained volunteers staff the
'phones, sited in offices some distance from the radio's studios.
They offer understanding listening, relevant information and, if
appropriate, advice on who should be approached for further help.
Except in extreme emergencies (if someone may be seriously at
risk of injury), the volunteers do not make referrals for help, but
encourage the callers to approach the appropriate agency. Records
are kept of calls received and, as confidentiality is an essential rule,
no one, other than staff of Family Care Line, is allowed access to
them.

　The paid staff of Family Care Line includes the regional Family
Network organiser, two full-time telephone counsellors to recruit
and train volunteers and administer the 'phone-in centre and a
project co-ordinator to deal with the broadcasting aspect. Apart
from the Family Network organiser, staff salaries are paid by
Picadilly Radio. The radio station also provides free advertising
(worth over £2,000 a week at commercial rates), office accommodation and contributes towards 'phone costs.

The public's response　In the first four months of Family Care
Line (May—August 1980) the lines were in almost continual use
and volunteers reported noticeable peaks of calls after each advertising trail. Over 2,000 calls were received in this time, with
marital and children's behaviour problems being most frequently
presented; each contributed about 10 per cent to the total number
of calls. People 'phoned with pregnancy worries and uncertainties
of how to get help from the health services. A member of the
project staff commented: 'Now the social texture is loosening, it
seems as though problems which people never dared speak about
are coming to the surface on our 'phone lines.' Volunteers'

training, support and the availability of quickly accessible sources of professional advice were stressed by the Family Network organiser as necessary with this type of case-load.

Radio programmes designed to meet callers' needs   For Piccadilly Radio, the 'phone links with families enables them to quickly see issues that worry people, for which public discussion and information is needed.   For instance, it became apparent that many listeners were tangled in 'step-relation' conflicts.   The Project Co-ordinator responded with a short studio discussion on 'step-problems' which included a volunteer role-playing a caller discussing step-parent worries.   The response was immediate and flooded the volunteers with families having similar problems.

Linking up callers — the start of local groups   Family Care Line demonstrates how new resources for family support can be mobilised within the community.   Piccadilly Radio beams out to a large but regionally defined population.   People who 'phone in and give their addresses can be located on a map and told about their local resources, including mutual-aid groups, to assist them. Following the 'step-problems' programme, callers were linked up with others who were going through similar experiences who were willing to offer mutual support in their area.   Family Network has thus helped establish several mutual-aid groups in areas of Greater Manchester.

In summary, the Child Care Switchboard and Family Care Line projects demonstrate the tremendous potential which local radio, linked to 'phone-in services, can offer to community health care by:

— reaching millions of homes to pass on information about health and health care
— enabling people to realise they are not alone with their problems, and thereby encouraging them to recognise their difficulties and to seek help
— linking people with health problems to appropriate sources of information and care
— acting like antenae, scanning huge populations and mapping out the changing patterns of families' health needs.   The image gained has great immediacy and is close to people's own perception of their needs, which may be different from that perceived by health professionals
— helping to establish networks of voluntary support and care for health, including mutual-aid groups

This type of social action broadcasting, in TV as well as radio, appears to be increasing in popularity with producers and the broadcasting companies. It must be emphasised, however, that without the generosity shown by the BBC and Piccadilly Radio towards the projects described above, this approach to community health care may be impossible.

In conclusion

It seems likely that the role of the voluntary sector in health care will receive increasing attention in the future. Mutual aid groups and other voluntary organisations concerned with health issues are expanding rapidly. Cuts in public expenditure in many statutory services are forcing a re-appraisal of the position of volunteers.

One lesson to emerge from the projects described in this chapter is that the voluntary sector has a certain contribution to make in developing more effective ways of delivering health care to families in particular situations. The special characteristics of the voluntary sectors' ways of working which are discussed here indicate that they can offer skills and experience which are different from those provided by the statutory and professional services. They provide complementary, rather than supplementary, resources.

Ways should be found to inform health professionals about the availability and strengths of the relevant voluntary organisations within their regions and districts so that their goodwill and expertise are used appropriately. In any such programme the inevitable limitations of these resources must also be emphasised. They are minute compared with the resources of the statutory services and should not be relied upon to make up for the deficiencies of government funding of the National Health Service.

It is also apparent from the study that the contribution of the voluntary sector to health care depends on a certain amount of financial security. Volunteers need to be prepared, supported and reimbursed for any expenses they incur; permanent staff need to be paid; funds should be available for the development of new ideas and to open up new areas of work. With the present cutbacks in the budgets of many health and local authorities, such support may be jeopardised. Joint Finance from health authorities and funding from central government departments may become increasingly important in the development of voluntary preventive health care schemes.

It looks as if the voluntary sector is a particularly rich source of innovation and creative experiments in the delivery of care. In this respect it often seems to outshine the statutory services. If this observation is correct it would be useful to find out why these differences exist and to consider how innovation in service delivery can be further promoted within the National Health Service. It is also important that those planning and managing the statutory services look for relevant innovation within the voluntary sector and consider how their own services could benefit from them.

Notes

1   This should be differentiated from the statutory sector, e.g. NHS and local authority services, the commercial profit-making sector, e.g. private health insurance companies, and the informal sector, e.g. relatives and friends.

2   Margaret Harrison, Home-Start Consultancy, 22 Princess Road West, Leicester LE1 6TP.

3   Volunteers working in the community should have insurance cover, particularly for public liability. For advice and information contact the Volunteer Centre, 29 Lower Kings Road, Berkhampsted, Herts, HP4 2AB. If volunteers are accountable to an employee of a health authority they are covered by that authority's indemnity. This will include volunteers working in the community as well as hospitals (HM (72) 6). But note: GPs are not health authority employees; health visitors, midwives and district nurses are usually. For further information about regulations concerning indemnity cover, contact your DHA Administrator or Personnel Officer.

4   Twins Clubs, 2 Steele Road, Chiswick, London W4.

5   The Stillbirth and Perinatal Death Association, 15a Christchurch Hill, London NW3 1JY.

6   Organisations for Parents Under Stress (OPUS), 26 Manor Drive, Pickering, Yorkshire.

7   Mrs Barbara Crowe, 19 Avenue Terrace, Westcliff-on-Sea, Essex SS0 7PL.

8   'The Loss of your Baby' can be obtained free from the Health Education Council, 78 New Oxford Street, London WC1A 1AH.

9   Available from OPUS, 2 Dagmar Grove, Alexandra Park, Nottingham.

10   This society is the local association of the National Society of Mentally Handicapped Children.

11   Although local authorities have a statutory duty to provide an adequate number of authorised sites for gypsies in their authorities, in 1982 in England there were enough sites for less than 50 per cent of gypsy caravans (Department of the Environment 1983). Thus about half the gypsy population have to live on illegal unauthorised sites from which they are likely to be evicted. These sites frequently lack the basic facilities for health, such as sanitation and clean water.

12   Kit Sampson, Mobile Health Clinic for Gypsy Families, Save the Children Fund, 17 Grove Lane, Camberwell, London SE5 8RD.

13   Available from Camera Talks Ltd, 31 North Row, London W1R 2EN.

14   For a description of volunteers' involvement in such broadcasting, see Community Service Volunteer's report 'C.S.V. and Social Action Broadcasting'. See also their training pack for beginners with broadcasting, entitled 'Local Radio Kit' and their 'Directory of Media Training Opportunities': all available from CSV, 237 Pentonville Road, London N1 9JT.

15   The National Children's Centre, Longroyd Bridge, Huddersfield, West Yorkshire.

16   Family Network, 35 Wilson Patten Street, Warrington, Cheshire WA1 1PG.

9 Working together for antenatal and pre-school health

Large resources are needed if every pregnant woman and pre-school child are to be reached with the necessary care, support and information for health. In previous chapters I have indicated the wealth of resources outside the NHS which is available to help achieve these goals: from the education and social services and from the voluntary sector. Many of the schemes I have described show the importance of partnerships between these agencies[1] and the health service: for training, for support and advice, for ideas about new ways of working and for the growth of trust. By working together we may be able to reshape our limited resources to be more acceptable and effective in reaching parents and young children in need of health care. But the need for collaboration is not confined to inter-agency contacts. Effective teamwork is also needed *within* each agency, between the different groups of workers. For instance, between community nurses and GPs and between the different levels of policy-makers, administrators, managers and fieldworkers. This chapter is concerned with ways in which the communities' resources may be brought together more effectively for maternity and child health. Collaboration within and between sectors of care for health is central to the WHO's strategy, 'Health For All by the Year 2000', to which this government is committed (WHO 1981). It featured prominently among the conclusions of the 1980 Commonwealth Health Ministers' meeting on Health and the Family (Commonwealth Health Ministers 1981).

Before discussing how collaboration may be developed, I will consider the objectives and problems of this approach to health care. Teamwork and collaboration are fashionable concepts which seem to have been accepted as conventional wisdom with little analysis or thought for the processes involved or the implications for all those involved. The case for a multi-agency approach in health care has to be justified. Bringing people together who normally work apart can be expensive in time, energy and money (Lonsdale, S. *et al.* 1980), and may be unpopular with groups of workers and organisations who see their scarce resources and hard-won identities threatened. And for the parents and children who are the focus of such services, there may be adverse consequences — for instance, in the confidentiality of certain information and the reduction in their choice of different systems of care.

The case for inter-agency collaboration for health in pregnancy, childhood or any time of life rests on the definition of health. If this is truly 'Everybody's Business' (DHSS 1976b) and the health services are seen within a spectrum of agencies for health promotion, as well as disease cures, then the need for collaboration is paramount.

That said, it is possible to outline some of the objectives of a collaborative approach for maternal and child health:

— to increase the availability of scarce resources by decreasing unnecessary overlap of function between agencies
— to improve the knowledge of other agencies' skills, roles and resources and thus to develop an informed and realistic baseline for collaboration. Such information should improve inter-agency referral. It might also bring a more coherent 'wholeness' to the various family services, helping families to find their way around them
— to improve the definition of families' health needs. Contributions from each of the statutory and voluntary agencies concerned with family care would emphasise the learning process of planning. It would also provide a broader vision of the resources available for health than is currently available
— to monitor the impact on families' health of policies and services which come from agencies outside the NHS. For instance, transport, income, housing and defence policies.

Each of these broad objectives can be translated at the national and local levels. The nature of my study leads me to concentrate on the latter.

However, the importance of the national level cannot be ignored. Government policies and practice, as well as those of powerful professional bodies, trade unions and voluntary organisations may frustrate or facilitate collaboration. Special ways may have to be found to promote co-ordinated policy and practice at this level: for instance the Childrens Committee (disbanded in 1981) or the suggested Independent Children's Council or Children's Congress (Deakin, N. 1982). It may be important to revive interest in the Central Policy Review Staff's proposals for a Joint Approach to Social Policy (1975) and the recommendations of the Black Report for inter-departmental collaboration on health-related policies at the cabinet level (Townsend, P. and Davidson, N. 1982).

But to return to the local scene. I will now outline some problems which threaten to confound the ideals of teamwork for health. They present, if you like, the unacceptable face of inter-agency collaboration.

— Between the local authority and health authority services there are major differences in management structure, ways of being financed, planning systems and timing of planning cycles, accountability and geographical boundaries (Rowbottom, R. and Hey, A. 1978). The professions within these services have different training, educational and social backgrounds and their ways of working and problem-solving vary greatly.

— To facilitate joint planning and work in areas of common concern to health and local authorities, various organisational structures and procedures have been introduced. These include Joint Consultative Councils, Joint Care Planning Teams, and Joint Finance (DHSS 1976a; 1977). There is evidence that these measures have not been particularly effective in promoting joint planning and development between local authority and health authority services (Norton, A. and Rogers, S. 1981).

— 'To be successful, rational planning requires a context where values are agreed and explicit, broad objectives can be agreed, information is complete and the tools for its analysis available and an environment which is relatively certain' (Norton, A. and Rogers, S. 1977). Evidence suggests that such a basis rarely exists either in local or health authorities. This undermines joint local health authority planning and confuses voluntary organisations trying to work with the statutory services (Leat, D. *et al.* 1981).

— The independent contractor status of GPs presents a further problem in joint planning with health and local authorities and voluntary groups. The organisation, financing and planning of general practice is separate and somewhat different from that of the primary health care services of health authorities (for instance health visitors and midwives). This can lead to poor channels of communication, misunderstandings and even resentment between all the different primary health care workers (Joint Working Group of the Standing Medical and Standing Nursing and Midwifery Advisory Committees 1981).

— The work of voluntary organisations embraces a wide range of needs which cut across the statutory services' divisions between health, education, housing and social services. Issues of representative democracy can also impede collaboration between the voluntary and statutory services. Local authorities, with their electoral accountability, may feel constrained in working closely with voluntary groups who have no such accountability.

— Collaboration between different agencies is often a negotiating and bargaining process. The different agencies look for advantages and financial gains which may come to them as a result of the collaboration. With the present resource constraints there are rarely any financial benefits which can be offered to 'buy' collaboration — anyway, in the long term.

These, then, are some of the problems which have to be overcome if the rhetoric exhorting us all to work together is to become a reality. Although major advances in joint agency planning and service development may require changes in the way the statutory services are structured, managed and financed, it would be wrong to overlook the less dramatic ways in which partnerships may be promoted, particularly at the operational and fieldworker level. The experience of this study is that the schemes which have succeeded in bringing groups of people together who normally work apart are often small-scale (not too many people or committees to consult with) and involve fieldworkers, rather than service managers or administrators (people closer to the needs of parents and children and further from the needs of the employing organisation). Although all these schemes have their own hallmark of individuality, certain common themes recur among them suggesting practical ways of overcoming the inherent difficulties in collaborative work between different agencies. For instance:

— special meetings and shared premises for the different statutory service and voluntary workers
— working in the same geographically defined communities
— special appointments for inter-agency liaison
— key personnel, who by the nature of their job may promote collaboration through their contacts with other agencies
— district and neighbourhood-based organisations for planning and developing services
— training programmes to develop appropriate knowledge, skills and attitudes for collaboration.

It is important to emphasise that this list is not meant to be exhaustive. Projects have been chosen to illustrate these six themes, though inevitably many of them reflect more than one theme.

I end with three projects which contain many key features of inter-agency and inter-disciplinary collaboration. Scope, Arbour and Family Start have each achieved radically new additions to their local services for family health by bringing together disciplines and agencies who usually work apart.

Shared premises

If agencies which normally work independently are to find ways of working together, personnel need opportunities to meet:

separate buildings and administrations can lock them into isolated networks of contacts.

Ariel, Barnsley

One way to increase contact between agencies is to encourage them to share premises and resources. This is illustrated by Ariel,[2] a community centre for self-help groups which has been initiated by a GP in his Barnsley practice. The centre aims to facilitate the development of self-help and voluntary groups and to promote partnerships between them and the primary health care team. It also acts as an information point where professionals, volunteers and members of the public can discover and locate local groups (Williamson, J. 1980).

At the start of the scheme the GP and several other local authority professionals contacted self-help groups and invited them to help set up the centre. They became its first members. As the centre has developed members have attempted to identify gaps in the local services and encouraged new groups to fill them. Membership is open to any local self-help group concerned with health or the social consequences of health problems, as well as other voluntary organisations working in the same field.

The contribution of the general practice to Ariel has been considerable. Member groups are offered, free of charge, meeting-rooms above the surgery, with projector facilities, and use of the practice's typewriter, duplicator and 'photocopier. They also have access to secretarial and administrative assistance, and professional advice from members of the health care team is available. Member groups contract to pay, at cost price, for expenses such as stationery, postage and telephone calls. They provide someone to help with Ariel's administration for one day every month. They also nominate one person to act as liaison officer between their organisation and the centre.

Ariel has member groups covering a wide range of health and social problems for all age groups. For families and young children there are self-help groups for parents of twins, mentally handi-capped and Downs Syndrome children, children with epilepsy and for parents at risk of child abuse.

Thatcham's Children's Centre

The possibility of increasing inter-agency collaboration by sharing common premises is also suggested by some of the child and family centres which have developed in recent years. Though these differ greatly in the way they are managed, in funding and the range of services they offer, all try to make the family the prime focus of their work. They bring together in one place partnerships of parents, volunteers and professionals from the health, education and social services.

In 1977 some mothers in Thatcham decided they needed a centre for the use of local mothers and children. Their concern was shared by the local GPs. At that time Thatcham had a population of about 8,000. By 1986 this figure was projected to increase to some 20,000. The new private estates were mainly composed of small two-bedroomed houses which attracted families with young children. After a few years, with the addition of extra children, these families moved on. By working on their own it seemed that health visitors, midwives, GPs and the providers of daycare in the area were only meeting a fraction of the parents' needs for support and care in these transient and isolated communities.

The first step in establishing the Children's Centre[3] was to gather together a group of local people who were enthusiastic about the idea and could contribute time and energy to its planning. A steering group was set up which included local mothers, the social services advisor for under-fives, a health visitor, a GP, the matron of the local children's home, the heads of the nearby infant and primary schools, and representatives from the Pre-school Playgroup Association, the toy library and the town and district council. Members of this group have been able to contribute an unusually wide range of skills, knowledge and resources to the centre's planning.

At the start of the project the district council leased the committee some common land on which they erected a prefabricated building. The centre, which has been given charitable status, opened in June 1980. Since then a playgroup has been held in one half of the building during weekdays. While this is running, the other half is used as a 'drop-in' centre for mothers with toddlers so they can have coffee, relax and meet other parents. During the rest of the week mother-and-toddler and postnatal support groups meet, with regular visits from health visitors and in addition, local midwives and a GP visit the postnatal support group. Health visitors and social workers have started a single parent support group, which meets regularly. A youth club for the under-twelves is held on two evenings a week and during the summer holidays there are play schemes. A local GP has started an evening health education programme for parents.

The paid staff of the centre include a playgroup supervisor and playgroup helpers. In addition a full-time supervisor is responsible for the parent's 'drop-in' sessions and for co-ordinating the activities of all the different groups using the centre. A voluntary youth leader helps run the youth club.

The capital cost of the initial stage of the project was some £32,000, which was met by grants from the town, district and county councils, private trusts, gifts from local firms and by many small fund-raising activities. The estimated annual revenue costs (1981) are about £7,000. Just over half this amount will be found by fund-raising activities and from the income of the playgroups and youth clubs held in the centre. It is hoped that the remaining sum will be met by grants from the local authority and other bodies.

There has been no formal evaluation of the success of this Children's Centre. However, the GP on the steering committee felt that the centre has already improved the working relationships between all the different professionals and volunteers working with families and young children in the area. Speaking from his own experience, he suggested that connections with all the different agencies involved in the centre were changing his own way of working, opening up new partnerships for sharing health information and care. In addition, his contacts with workers from many different disciplines were introducing him to new ideas and possibilities for providing a more complete form of family care in pregnancy and early childhood. He was now aware of many more community resources for health care.

Working in the same geographically defined populations

The co-ordination of maternity and pre-school services from local and health authorities and from the voluntary sector of care may be facilitated if they all work within a common population.

The Barclay Report (1982) recommended the development of community-based social work, suggesting that valuable voluntary and informal caring resources may be wasted if professionals work with isolated individuals rather than with whole communities (see chap. 7). The Acheson Committee on Primary Health Care in Inner London (1981) and the Joint Working Group of the Standing Medical, Nursing and Midwifery Advisory Committees (1981) both recognised that in inner urban areas there may be a particular need for primary health care workers to cover an entire population in a defined neighbourhood. They point to the inefficiency of working arrangements which result in workers from many different general practices visiting the same street and even the same block of flats. This type of service organisation makes communication between different workers difficult and time-consuming. The Acheson Report recommended that groups of GPs should be encouraged:

> to concentrate their practice areas so as to facilitate close working relationships with other primary care workers. The health and local authorities should, as a matter or priority,

ensure that the organisation of the working areas of other members of the primary care team are parallel to those of the GPs.   (para 5.13)

The Acheson Committee and the Joint Working Group suggested that in some urban areas it might be advantageous for the health visiting services to revert from being GP-attached to working within geographically defined communities — as most of them did pre-1960. Since then government policy has encouraged a type of organisation known as 'GP attachment' in which health visitors' case loads are limited to the patients on GPs' lists. Patients may be scattered over large areas which, in urban areas, often overlap with the areas covered by other GPs. About 90 per cent of health visitors now work in this way (Dunnell and Dobbs 1982).

What follows describes an experiment in the 'detachment' of health visitors and district nurses from GPs which may have relevance to some other urban areas. It is important, however, to note the comment of the Acheson Report (1981) 'The absence of attachment does not necessarily exclude the possibility of team-work any more than the presence of an attachment scheme guarantees its existence' (para 5.3).

Barnsley Area Health Authority

On 1 January, 1979, the health visitors and district nurses of Barnsley Area Health Authority changed from GP attachment to working in geographically defined neighbourhoods.[4] The discussions leading to this decision revealed that health visitors and district nurses felt that GP attachment had complicated their liaison with midwives and social workers who worked in geographical zones; and that it diminished their effectiveness in their local communities, with whom they were no longer closely identified. Nursing officers, aware of the need to save money, pointed to the time spent travelling to reach families scattered over large areas of Barnsley. For the families themselves the attachment of community nurses to GPs sometimes meant that they dealt with one health visitor in the home, another in the clinic and yet another in the school. Because of the overlap of GPs' attachment areas, this resulted in an excessive number of community nurses visiting the same neighbourhood and often even the same street (Barnsley Area Health Authority 1978).

When the health visitors and district nurses reverted to working in geographically defined zones, these were carefully chosen to coincide with those in which the midwives and social workers worked. They approximated, as closely as possible, with the neighbourhoods of the health visitors' former GP practices. In this way it was hoped to maximise the liaison with the midwifery and social services while minimising the disruption experienced by GPs at the time of the reorganisation. Great care was taken to consult with GPs before these changes were made.

Reports from the health authority suggest that the reorganised service has certain advantages for the co-ordination of work between the community nurses, midwives, social workers and parents in the community (Barnsley Area Health Authority 1979). Direct contact between health visitors, district nurses, midwives and social workers was reported to be greatly increased, with a resultant increase in the transfer of information relevant to their work. This improved liaison was partly because, with the exception of the social workers, they all now shared a common building. Communication between these different workers was also made easier by the decrease in the number of people with whom each of them worked. For instance, in the neighbourhood of Athersley the number of health visitors dropped from fifteen, under the GP-attachment scheme, to three. The number of district nurses dropped from ten to two.[5] The health visitors and district nurses reported that they were gradually becoming a recognisable part of their local communities, which helped them in their preventive work and gave them more job satisfaction. With the exception of two areas, health visitors dealt with the whole family at home, clinic and school.

At the start of the scheme, reports from GPs were less favourable. Although the reorganisation was designed to minimise their problems, those with widely scattered patients now had to deal with several health visitors and district nurses instead of just one or two. To overcome this difficulty, GPs were given the names of key liaison nursing officers whom they could contact if they had trouble finding a patient's community nurse.

The change in health visitors' way of working has been accompanied by an increase in the number of people visited at home and a decrease in the mileage travelled (see table 3). Between 1978 and 1980 there were no significant alterations in the numbers of health visiting staff in post or any other major changes in the health visiting service or in the population structure in the area of Barnsley AHA which could account for these differences. It seems, therefore, that in Barnsley this type of reorganised community nursing service is enabling more of their resources to reach a greater proportion of the population.

It will be important to examine the wider implications of this change — for instance its effects on the work of GPs and on the health of the community.

Table 3: *Barnsley AHA health visiting 1977-1980*

	1977	1978*	1979	1980	% change since 1978	
					1979	1980
No. of persons seen at least once						
0—5 years	8,643	8,402	10,649	11,428	+27	+36
All ages	17,268	16,262	22,140	26,267	+36	+62
Total effective home visits						
All ages	41,886	47,655	56,657	79,654	+19	+67
HVs total mileage	103,082	102,341	68,415	74,478	-33	-28
Miles per effective home visit	2.5	2.2	1.2	0.9	-44	-58

*HVs changed from GP-attachment to geographical patchwork on 1.1.79.

Special appointments for inter-agency liaison

The creation within health and local authorities of appointments with a responsibility for inter-agency liaison may help to develop and co-ordinate maternity and pre-school services across departmental and professional boundaries.   To varying degrees such appointments invest the relevant officers with power to influence their own services' planning and to have access to resources to develop collaborative ways of working with other agencies. The extent to which the holders of these appointments can succeed in their role probably depends on factors such as their personality, communication skills, political sensitivity, status and the benefits which other organisations can gain from working with them.

I will refer only to special appointments for liaison work between the health service and the voluntary sector. However, within health authorities and departments of social services there are also officers with special responsibilities for liaison between departments such as the social services.   The project concerning homeless families in Westminster (chap. 2) is an example of the collaborative project which may result from the work of these officers.

The first appointment in the health service for liaison and development work with the voluntary sector was made in 1963. The majority of Voluntary Service Co-ordinators (VSCs) are funded by health authorities. Most are based in hospitals and are concerned with co-ordinating the work of volunteers and voluntary organisations in this institutional situation (Volunteer Centre 1976). For instance, VSCs may help to establish play schemes in hospital antenatal clinics. But recently, attention has turned to the expanding role of volunteers in primary health care teams, for instance in Norwich, Medway and South Hammersmith Health Districts. I will describe some aspects of the latter scheme's development.

A health-centre-based voluntary service co-ordinator

In 1979 a VSC was appointed to work in Milson Road Health Centre in South Hammersmith Health District.[6] The first and second years' funding for this new post came respectively from the budgets of Joint Finance and the Inner Area Programme. At that time this 4-year-old health centre had approximately 11,000 registered patients and a large number of staff including, among others, four GPs, fifteen district nurses, five health visitors, a social worker and eight administrators.

The health centre serves an inner city area where the unbalanced outward migration of working-aged people was thought to have destroyed many of the natural family and informal neighbourhood support systems for mothers and young children and the elderly. It was hoped that the VSC would be able to identify and support those sources of informal and voluntary care which still existed, develop new ones and help integrate the work of volunteers with that of the primary health care team. In particular, one of the initial aims of the project was to facilitate the care available to mothers with difficult pregnancies and those with new babies. The VSC would recruit and support volunteers who would work closely with the midwife and health visitors. They would offer a befriending service with practical help in attending clinics and in generally coping with the new demands of parenthood.

The Voluntary Organisations Research Unit of the Policy Studies Institute monitored the development and growth of this project in the first year (Morcroft, I. 1981). Their report is a useful account of the problems which this type of worker may face when first joining a health centre. Initially the VSC felt isolated and had difficulty in being accepted by members of the primary health care team who did not appear to understand the role of volunteers. Many of the health service staff, though not decrying volunteers, saw them as peripheral or even irrelevant in their work. They were concerned about their accountability (chap. 8) should anything go wrong when a volunteer was working with a patient. The task of volunteer development in this setting was therefore slow. Gradually, however, the VSC and the volunteers were able to show even the most sceptical members of the staff the potential which lay in the volunteer/professional partnership in primary health care.

In this South Hammersmith project many of these initial problems of acceptance were probably related to the haste with which the project had to start as short-term funding suddenly became available. The speed with which the bloc grant had to be taken up curtailed the important period of pre-project consultation between members of the primary health care team and those setting up the project. This led to confusion among members of the team about the aims of the project and the role and scope of the work of the VSC and volunteers. In turn, the organisers themselves may not have fully appreciated the way in which the health care team worked and the importance of involving more than a GP in planning the project. It may be relevant to note how similar these problems of acceptance of a new team member are to those reported when health visitors were first attached to general practices (Ambler *et al.* 1968; Arin, J. 1968).

Key personnel, whose jobs may promote collaboration

Many of the schemes and service developments already described suggest that among the fieldworkers of the various statutory and voluntary agencies there are individuals with unusual degrees of motivation, skill and knowledge for collaborative work. Unlike the special appointments described in the previous section, these people have no particular responsibility for playing a liaison role: they seem to take it on as part of their everyday work. These are, if you like, the services' natural agents for bringing people together and developing ways of working across departmental boundaries. People who have the skills to do this have been called 'reticulists' (Friend *et al.* 1974). It may be important to recognise these workers as a special group so that their talents and motivation can be supported and given opportunities for development. To do this we need to know far more about the way in which these attributes can be identified and developed.

The position of general practice

The type of job which facilitates these fieldworkers' abilities to work in this way may also be important. It seems, for instance, that some jobs provide particularly advantageous positions in the community for making contact and establishing trust and respect with a wide range of different care-giving agencies. The special position of general practitioners for facilitating and bringing together partnerships of different people for the support of parents in pregnancy and in early childhood has already been mentioned (see pp. 32, 82). A few other multi-agency projects, wholly or partly initiated by GPs, should also be mentioned. For instance, in Sheffield[7] some GPs have encouraged an English-as-a-second-language playgroup to run from their practice. This is for local parents and children whose first language is not English. The GPs consider this playgroup as an integral part of total family health care in this depressed city area. In London a GP and child psychologist[8] have established a scheme which offers support to mothers in the practice having their first baby, with the help of volunteers who are patients of the practice. The project has become a focus for a co-ordinated approach to pregnancy and postnatal care in the health centre.

The position of health visitors

Like GPs, health visitors have the type of job which may provide them with the necessary contacts to establish partnerships with workers in the other statutory services. In addition, they are in a unique position to develop new ways of working with the voluntary and informal sector of family care in their neighbourhoods. This is indicated by the large number of parent self-help support groups which have been partly or wholly initiated and supported by health visitors. I heard of many of these, including numerous postnatal and breast-feeding groups and mother-and-toddler clubs. Some of them appear to be successful in attracting regular attendance from parents living in stressful and depriving situations (Chapman, S. and Reynolds, E. 1982; Palfreeman, S. 1982).

The account below comes from a health visitor in Harrow:[9]

In 1969 some mothers with small children in a middle-class area of Harrow expressed a need for small postnatal support groups. These young mothers felt they would prefer small, more intimate groups to large postnatal support groups run from clinics. Many of them had worked in early pregnancy in interesting jobs, and were lonely and depressed after the arrival of their first babies. Many did not have relations living near, or had husbands whose jobs took them away from home.

Gradually we were able to bring together eight to ten mothers with young children, who lived within walking distance of each other, to form a group. The means of contact was through health visitors, GPs and social workers, and the only criterion was that the mother was lonely and had a baby or small child to care for.

To overcome the breakdown of the extended family and provide 'artificial' aunts, uncles and cousins for the children, each member took it in turn to hold the meeting in her own home. As most of the houses were fairly large, eight to ten mothers and children could easily be accommodated, but when many of the mothers had another baby within two or three years, it was difficult to find room for the increase in the number of children. Children who were aged two years and under when they entered related easily to each other as they grew, but we found that children who entered between the ages of three to five years were more easily bored and disruptive at group meetings.

Before each group was formed a leader would be chosen. The qualities we looked for were calmness, common sense, experience with people and, if possible, some experience with children.   Some former professional people such as social workers, teachers and probation officers became leaders, but most leaders had had no previous experience of leading a group.

At first I helped the new leaders to start their groups, but as time went on the more experienced leaders would help new leaders set up groups.   Experienced leaders then became advisers.

There are now 28 groups in the Borough, comprising a complete cross-section of social class. Each group is of less than five years duration and has six to eight mothers.   Another ten groups are of between five and ten years duration, some of whose members have moved too far away to attend regularly but still keep in touch and meet occasionally.

Many new ideas have been tried in the last three years but the basic plan is the same as it was ten years ago.   Six groups now form a unit, so that up to 36 people are quite closely in touch with each other and have, on several occasions, hired halls for parties or arranged nearly-new or toy sales, fêtes and autumn fairs.   The mothers have chosen the name CHAT (contact, health and teaching) for the overall title of the groups.   Each group is known by a number and each unit by a letter.   All CHAT members are invited to all social events so the mothers with small children have the opportunity of making a large circle of friends.

An eight week course is organized once a year from a local clinic, with a different speaker each week on some aspect of health or education from the baby to the teenage child, and all CHAT members are invited.   A crèche is run in conjunction with the course by a nursery nurse tutor, students from a local college and students from a sixth form college.

Our library of 130 books on all aspects of child development and community life was brought together through voluntary effort and each group has five books for two or three months before they are circulated again.   Many of these books give insight into community problems and activities and after being group members for about a year, many CHAT families have started some work in the community. In the past some members have taught parentcraft to teenage boys and girls taking a Family and Community course (CSE mode 3) at a comprehensive school.

We found that each group can usually support one member

with deeper problemś, such as depression or rejection of her baby, and the supported mother usually improves rapidly; in such cases I keep closely in touch with the mother's GP.

(Hiskins, G. 1981)

At the time of writing these postnatal support groups are the subject of an evaluation by an independent observer as part of the SSRC Pre-school Evaluation Project, Bristol University.

The position of health education officers: Newpin

The Unit for the Study of Health Policy (1979) suggested that Health Education Officers (HEOs) could have a key role in developing multi-agency approaches to community health care. Some HEOs are using their position to do this, bringing together different types of services to identify and develop ways of meeting the health needs of parents in pregnancy and their children's early years of life.

The project 'Newpin' (New Parent Infant Network)[10] in Southwark illustrates this. It has developed within a community which has all the hallmarks of inner city deprivation — poverty, high unemployment, poor housing, and frequent moves for the families living in it. The health visitors, paediatricians and others working in the area report a high incidence of isolation and depression in women when they are pregnant and bringing up young children, often on their own. Not surprisingly, there tends to be an above-average incidence of early childhood death and preventable illness and disability, including that caused by child abuse.

Before the start of Newpin, it seems that many of the health and social workers in the district were frustrated by their inability, when working alone, to provide the type of support and care which many families needed. Too often they picked up the pieces after the crises, perhaps in the casualty department or the case conference.

Recognising the need for a preventive approach to these problems the District Health Education Officer looked for ways of mobilising new resources for family care in the community and new ways of working. In 1979 she organised a series of multi-disciplinary meetings to which she invited the community paediatrician, health visitors, midwives, officers of the social services, the Community Health Council and local voluntary agencies such as the Pre-school Playgroups Association, the National Childbirth Trust and Parents Anonymous. This was the beginning of a forum in which families' difficulties could be examined from different perspectives. Gradually, the idea of Newpin evolved.

Some three years after these initial discussions, Newpin is a registered charity employing a full-time co-ordinator (a former health visitor from the district) and a full-time secretary. The project has a permanent base in a health authority building in the community, as well as accommodation in Guy's Hospital's child health clinic.

The main objective of Newpin is to provide voluntary support by local mothers to families during pregnancy and children's early life, which is continued while there is need. Much of the co-ordinator's work is concerned with recruiting volunteers, training them, matching them with suitable families who need visiting and supporting the volunteers themselves in their work and their own development.

An executive committee is responsible for the project's planning and development and the support of the project team. This committee is composed of the District HEO, the community paediatrician, a senior nursing officer, the social services officer responsible for child abuse cases and an officer from the National Childbirth Trust. A research programme has been established to monitor the project's work.

Though the project is still only in its infancy, several observations are worth noting. The first is that, in the view of its originator, it has taken far longer to establish than she had originally envisaged. People have to be persuaded into ways of working which are relatively untested and untried.

There are also financial problems. The annual estimate of the project's cost is about £21,000. At the start of the scheme National Westminster Enterprises (of the National Westminster Bank) seconded, with no charge, a full-time member of their staff to act as an appeals secretary. Since then fund-raising has been done by a member of the trustees in his spare time. So far, no grant has been received from either the health or local authority, despite the relevance of the project to their work. This story is typical of many I heard.

And finally there is the question of the support and continuing education of the volunteers themselves. The need for this has proved greater than was originally anticipated. The co-ordinator commented that this was probably because the project is drawing its volunteers from an inner city community whose members would not normally have the confidence or educational experience to consider themselves as potential volunteers. This observation is reminiscent of other schemes which I have described — for instance Home-Start (see chap. 8). It seems that if volunteering is to move out of its traditional middle-class domain, issues of volunteer preparation, support and continuing education are of crucial importance. Their financial implications should not be under-estimated by grant-giving bodies.

District and neighbourhood-based organisation for planning and developing services

Many of the collaborative schemes described so far might be called 'once-off' attempts to solve particular local problems. They have usually arisen from the vision and energy of a few highly committed individuals or agencies whose concern about certain problems happen to coincide. Characteristically these schemes have not developed as a result of an overall planning and development strategy for the maternity or pre-school services for the whole district or neighbourhood.

Although it is important to encourage this type of individual response to local need, isolated innovations may be a wasteful way of moving forward. For the providers of maternity and pre-school services these innovations can result either in duplication or underutilisation of resources. For the users they may produce a confusing array of poorly co-ordinated or even conflicting options for care.

Local planning and advisory structures are required for antenatal and pre-school care which can take an overall view of the needs of the district and provide a forum in which all those concerned can contribute. It is relevant to recall the message of the Rt Hon. Patrick Jenkin (then Secretary of State for Social Services) when writing to the chairmen and members of the new district health authorities: 'local initiatives, local decisions and local responsibility is what we want to encourage . . . You therefore have a wider opportunity than your predecessors to plan and develop the services in the light of local needs and circumstances' (DHSS 1981a).

A variety of structures are available to play this type of role. Joint consultative councils and joint care planning teams, which bridge the gap between health and local authorities, have already been mentioned. Health authorities' district planning teams advise the district management teams on the planning of services for particular client groups (e.g. children) or particular services (e.g. maternity). These teams may include representatives from local authority services, community health councils and voluntary bodies. A national survey in 1978 showed that 44 per cent of districts and single district areas had such teams for the maternity services. Sixty-six per cent had teams for children's services (Muller *et al.* 1981).

The Maternity Services Advisory Committee (1982) has proposed that a new type of multidisciplinary planning group should be established in each district, known as the Maternity Services Liaison Committee. This will attempt to

ensure integration between the specialist and the community

maternity services. Each Committee should have two functions, the agreement of generally applicable procedures and the monitoring of the effectiveness of procedures as they apply to the individual woman.   (para. 1.13)

It seems therefore that these committees will be concerned mainly with the medical/clinical aspects of pregnancy care. It is suggested, however, that for some parts of their work, lay membership[11] may be desirable.

But planning and development groups to consider the broad spectrum of services which concern antenatal and pre-school health in a locality need not originate from the health services. For instance, several types of co-ordinating groups have been initiated by local authority social services and education departments.

The proliferation of these groups in recent years probably reflects the previous policy of the DHSS and DES (1976; 1978) to encourage the co-ordination of local services for children under five. Against these developments there seems a striking absence of similar local schemes for the co-ordination of maternity care (Dowling, S. forthcoming).

Local groups for good practices in antenatal health

One exception comes from the National Council for Voluntary Organisations,[12] which has recently introduced a scheme to establish groups to study and disseminate information about local good practices in antenatal health. Early in 1983 groups were started in Manchester,[13] Sheffield[14] and South Tees.[15] This initiative is modelled on the International Hospital Federations Scheme for 'Good practices in mental health' (Gordon, P. 1980). Like the mental health projects, the maternity study groups aim to bring together many of those with health interests and skills in maternity care in the local area. These include people from the voluntary sector as well as the different statutory services. The experience of the 'Good practices in mental health' scheme has been that the local projects have often become a focus for improving inter-agency collaboration and the joint development of services.

Local pre-school co-ordinating groups: Liverpool's POC

Let me return to the pre-school co-ordinating groups. In many parts of the country these are now well established and may be useful models for the promotion of collaborative planning for many different client groups. A national survey of local authority procedures for co-ordinating the statutory and voluntary services for the under-fives has shown the variety of structure, representation and function within these groups (Bradley, M. 1982). The impression gained from their experience is that an effective type of organisation may be one which attempts to knit together the four different levels of local services:

— families who use the services
— fieldworkers (statutory and non-statutory)
— managers of the statutory services
— councillors and members of health authorities.

Liverpool's Pre-school Organisations Committee (POC)[16] was established in 1976 to co-ordinate pre-school voluntary work in Liverpool. It was also asked to recommend to a social services committee of the local authority ways in which grants should be allocated to voluntary groups. In this latter function, POC is probably unique among pre-school co-ordinating committees. In the year 1980/81 the committee was concerned with the distribution of just over £41,000 in grants from social services, Urban Aid and the Inner City Partnership Fund.

POC meets regularly in the city council's committee rooms and receives its secretarial and administrative services from the social services' department. When POC was first set up, the health services were not represented in the group. Their membership was invited in 1979 after it became apparent that many voluntary groups were requesting more support and contact with the health services. Other members of POC include officers from departments of social services, education and the city solicitors, together with a large representation from local voluntary groups, such as Save the Children Fund, the Liverpool Playgroup Action Committee, the National Association for the Welfare of Children in Hospital, Homelink, Liverpool Council for Voluntary Services and Liverpool Parents' and Toddler's Association. In addition, individuals with special skills and knowledge relevant to the work of the committee are co-opted when necessary.

The secretary of POC describes three levels at which they work. At one level POC attempts to influence the senior managers and policy-makers responsible for the different statutory pre-school services. To this end they have developed liaison and personal contacts with the senior officers of the local authority services and the health authority. Whenever necessary they lobby members of the health authority, councillors and their MPs. Recommendations arising from POC meetings are referred on to the appropriate local authority committees.

At another level, POC supports local pre-school voluntary organisations and groups — for instance with funds, equipment, training and information. The free newspaper *Roundabout*, financed by POC, contains information about different pre-school groups, services and parents. It is distributed widely through child health clinics, playgroups, childminders, mother-and-toddler groups and day nurseries.

The third part of POC's work concerns the identification of parents' and children's needs and their ideas and views about the various services provided. In this respect the wide representation of voluntary groups and parents on the committee is important. In 1976/7, they surveyed households in five areas of Liverpool to find the type of pre-school care parents wanted for their children. Their report was used by the city council when developing its pre-school policies (Bradley, M. and Kucharski, R. 1977).

The success of POC may perhaps be gauged by its increasing involvement in pre-school initiatives in Liverpool and its continued funding. Some of these initiatives are of particular relevance to the health services: they have assisted a local GP who set up mother-and-toddler groups with a focus on health and education and they have attempted to introduce play into the hospital antenatal clinics.

In the latter example the committee was responding to repeated representations from their community health council and other groups about the lack of facilities for children in these clinics. They offered the health authority £1,000 from their budget towards play equipment. They also suggested that voluntary play staff from the National Association for the Welfare of Children in Hospital and the National Childbirth Trust would be prepared to assist in supervising children's play. As there was little room to establish play facilities in the clinics, POC offered to provide a small Portacabin close to the clinic. This was to be installed, free of charge, by Community Industry, a youth training scheme. Unfortunately it has not proved possible to find a suitable site, so POC have had to change their plans: they are now equipping and providing toy boxes and book libraries in each of the clinics.

Training programmes

So far I have tended to highlight apparently successful partnerships between health, local authority and voluntary agencies. It would be misleading, however, not to register that I also heard of failures. It seems that organisational arrangements for inter-agency collaboration are not enough. The attitudes, skills and knowledge of those working in such partnerships are also important.

Studies of inter-professional work show widespread ignorance about the training, roles and skills of other professions; also about the structure and nature of the organisations in which they work (Hallett, C. and Stevenson, O. 1980). Research into inter-professional work in primary health care teams and with child-abuse cases indicates how inadequate knowledge about other professions may lead to negative and even hostile attitudes towards them. This may result in a failure in trust and a reluctance to share information, even when this is essential — for instance with suspected child abuse (Bruce, N. 1980). 'Though there is little evidence on multi-agency work involving volunteers, it appears that here there are also problems of inappropriate attitudes and ignorance about the experience and skills they can contribute (Leat, D. *et al.* 1981).

Training programmes for those involved in multi-agency work have been suggested as a way of ameliorating these problems (Hallet, C. and Stevenson, O. 1980). Perhaps it was surprising, therefore, that I identified relatively few attempts to teach skills and knowledge which may facilitate inter-agency collaboration. Those which I did encounter are described below. They are divided into programmes which operate at a national and regional level and those which are designed specifically for local workers.

Training at a national and regional level

Joint meetings of professional training bodies   During the last ten years some of the professional training bodies have met regularly to try and further the development of multi-disciplinary training. They have included the Council for the Training of Health Visitors (later the Council for the Education and Training of Health Visitors), the Royal College of General Practitioners, the National Institute for Social Work, the Central Council for the Education and Training of Social Workers and the Panel of Assessors for District Nurse Training.

Together these training bodies have organised a series of educational events for multi-disciplinary groups of health visitors, GPs, social workers and district nurses (Flack, G.1977; England, H. 1980). Resulting from these a steering group was set up in 1980, composed of representatives of the four disciplines. It aims to establish ways in which multi-disciplinary training can be introduced into different parts of each profession's training. Another outcome of this joint initiative has been the production of a collection of exercises for multi-disciplinary training (Griffiths, K. *et al.* 1979).

Multi-agency work as part of professionals' basic training   There appears to be little evidence on the extent to which skills for inter-agency collaboration are taught in the basic training courses of the different professions. It seems that such teaching may be more common in health visitor and social work courses than among those of medical students. In the author's medical school a variety of multi-disciplinary workshops have been introduced in the undergraduate community medicine course as well as other parts of the clinical course.[17] Students of medicine, health visiting, district nursing, social work and education, together with volunteers, take part in small-group exercises. They examine their roles and skills in managing different types of family problems, such as child abuse or childhood disability. Exercises have been devised to help students learn from each other about their different backgrounds and education and the way these may manifest themselves when working in multi-agency teams.

Post-basic multi-professional course in pre-school work   A report by the Voluntary Organisations Liaison Committee for the Under Fives (VOLCUF) in 1977 recommended that there should be a foundation course to teach the skills and knowledge necessary for multi-agency work in the pre-school field. Two such courses have now been established: a two-year part-time evening course at Roehampton Institute of Higher Education and a one-year sandwich course at the School of Applied Social Studies, Bristol University. They are both for professionally qualified staff from the health, social work and education services. The Bristol course also takes candidates from the voluntary sector.

Locally based training: Hampshire-based study project

Courses which draw their participants from a local area have certain advantages over these national and regional courses. They may be based within districts or the catchment areas of general practices, schools or clinics. In these environments, the different agencies involved can develop their collaborative skills and knowledge in the context of real, rather than hypothetical, working situations.   Such training initiatives, in addition to their educational functions, can contribute to the development and planning of local services and the definition of families' needs.

This dual function of training and service development is particularly well illustrated in the Hampshire-based study project.[18] This was a six-month educational experiment aimed to increase and improve collaboration between all groups providing pre-school care in six different neighbourhoods throughout Hampshire county. As well as studying the different ways in which professionals and volunteers in the pre-school field worked, the study groups were intended to explore the needs of local families and identify problems and gaps in the services which might require attention either at the fieldworker or managment level (Poulton, G. and Campbell, G. 1979). The project was approved by the joint care planning team. Money for tutors' fees and secretarial help was obtained from the joint funding budget of the health authority. The University of Southampton's Departments of Sociology and Social Administration and Education were jointly responsible for developing and administering the study project in close liaison with officers from the relevant departments of the local authority.

The first three of the evening meetings were held at the university at weekly intervals. Practitioners and research workers were invited to present new research findings concerning the pre-school services. Project members were then divided into six neighbourhood study groups. These met six times at fortnightly intervals within their local area. Written and verbal reports of each group's progress and findings were fed back to the other groups halfway through the project and again at the end.

Each of the six study groups was centred on a neighbourhood which coincided, as far as possible, with the local administrative unit of the health or local authority services. The group members worked within this neighbourhood and were fieldworkers, rather than service managers. Among the fifty-eight project workers recruited throughout the county there were health visitors, clinical medical officers, social workers, community workers, teachers, playgroup organisers, education welfare officers, and the co-ordinator of Scope (see page 144). University tutors with experience in group work led the groups.

The final report of the project describes the findings of the six study groups, and much of it is relevant to health visitors and doctors as well as to the managers of the health service. It was suggested, for instance, that in neighbourhoods where there was a high turnover of health visitors and social workers, regular lists of these staff in post should be provided for line managers and field-workers; also that there should be a manual listing staff structures, areas of responsibility of the different workers and outlining the procedures adopted within each agency.

The report was submitted to the senior officers of each of the relevant services and to the joint care planning team. It was hoped that as they had supported the scheme, they would comment and respond to the findings and recommendations of the groups. Only one reply was received.

Despite this disappointing response from the statutory service managers, the fieldworkers tried to ensure that the experience of this short experiment was not lost. They therefore set up their own groups (called 'Educare' groups) in different parts of the county and organised local programmes.

The report of this project contains many useful tips for anyone wanting to set up a similar study exercise. For instance, if the study groups were drawn from too large a catchment area it seemed that the group members could not relate to specific neighbourhood problems. Their discussions tended to be too general in nature. The project organisers thought that the provision of a written record of each group's work was a useful way of making them focus their discussions. However, it seems that this may have inhibited some members who were aware that the reports would ultimately be seen by their managers. Records of these group discussions indicated that playgroup organisers and advisers and community workers were particularly useful in contributing information on local patterns of family services. The timing of the sessions in the evenings probably inhibited the attendance of fieldworkers with young children.

Three schemes in detail

I conclude this chapter with descriptions of three examples of the way in which resources for health may be reshaped when different agencies and groups of workers develop partnerships of planning and service provision for local families. These schemes, from Southampton, Liverpool and Oldham have achieved an unusual degree of teamwork and illustrate further many of the points I have already discussed in relation to inter-agency collaboration. Each has achieved radically new additions to the existing local services for pregnancy and the pre-school years. This has been done by pooling the experience of several disciplines and sectors of care, by the careful definition of family needs and the matching of skills and resources to meet these needs. By rethinking and remoulding their approach to care in pregnancy and early childhood, the schemes have all succeeded in reaching groups of parents and young children whom the statutory health and social services find elusive. In short, the experience of Scope, Arbour, and Family Start show that, in certain circumstances, the services of a carefully planned collaborative scheme can be more extensive and more appropriate for the needs of families than those provided by individual agencies working on their own.

Scope, Southampton[19]

Scope is a network of neighbourhood support groups for women with pre-school children. At the time of writing (1981), these groups cover some ten neighbourhoods of Southampton. Most of them are on postwar council estates where women often bring up their children in stressful home circumstances, with little previous experience of childrearing and minimal support from friends or relatives. Research has suggested that, as a group, Scope families have an above average risk of ill-health and a particular need for health information and care (Hevey, D. and Jackson, S. 1982).

Aims and objectives   It is difficult to attribute the development of Scope to any one discipline or sector of family care. Certainly the influence of education — both early childhood and adult education — has been strong. The two originators of the project are well known for their work in the field of community education and for helping to establish the first Educational Home Visiting Scheme in this country in Yorkshire (Smith, G. 1975; see also chap. 6 page 75). Yet the objectives of Scope and the way in which it operates can also be seen in the context of preventive health. It provides parents with information about health and child development, and also gives emotional and practical support to relieve some of the stress of childrearing. This type of social support may be an important influence on the health of parents and children.

The project also aims to help people use the health and other statutory services appropriately and to their maximum benefit.

> Our experience in Scope over the past four years suggests that a great need exists for people who use statutory services to be able to present clear, specific requests for help at the correct point in the system. In such a process the individuals concerned need guidance and support. When appropriate instances arise, members can, and do, receive help in approaching a particular part of the services. More importantly, the work in groups encourages members to gain sufficient confidence and knowledge of the services to make their own approaches. It also follows that greater knowledge and confidence in themselves will reduce demands by people who have become dependent on the services. (Poulton, G. and Cousins, L. 1980)

Much of the following account is based on information from the annual reports of Scope which have carefully documented each stage of the project's development (Poulton, G. 1977; Poulton G. 1978; Poulton, G. 1979; Poulton and Cousins, L. 1980). For a more detailed account of Scope's work, readers are referred to the Report of the SSRC Pre-School Project from which the following introduction to the project's work is taken.

> Groups of 6 to 12 women meet weekly in any convenient local premises, such as schools, clinics and church halls. A crèche is provided for the children in the same or an adjacent room and the mothers engage in group discussions on issues of relevance to them. Problems relating to health, child development and management and personal relationships are among the most frequently chosen topics. As a matter of principle, there is no charge for participation.
>
> The groups are convened by volunteers who have normally been group members for some time and have, in addition, taken

part in an informal training course. There are usually two convenors per group, one of whom acts as crèche leader. Convenors claim an expenses allowance of £3.00 per week to cover incidental items such as bus fares to and from training sessions, phone calls etc.

At the centre of the network is the SCOPE Co-ordinator, who is the single professional worker co-ordinating all its activities . . . In addition, small payments are made for an assistant co-ordinator and for some secretarial/administrative assistance.

SCOPE now operates a Family Centre providing short term residential breaks for families experiencing particular stress. The Family Centre provides a central focus for the network of groups, a readily available contact point for the co-ordinator and a base for wider activities.

(Hevey, D. and Jackson, S. 1982)

Funding   In 1978/79 and 1979/80 the annual cost of Scope was about £9,000. Funding has been acquired from various sources: Barclays Bank, the health and local authorities and local industry.

The families   Parents join Scope groups from a variety of sources. Some are invited by active group members, while others are asked by health visitors, social workers and other fieldworkers. If referred by a professional the parents always have full knowledge of the referral and are asked if they agree to a visit at home by the co-ordinator. Confidentiality is a prime consideration. As a matter of policy, Scope keeps no records of referrals other than their names and addresses. In the year 1979/80, one hundred and ninety-four families were referred to Scope, this figure representing nearly a threefold increase in referrals since the year 1977/78. Of the referrals in 1979/80, 58 per cent came from health visitors.

On receiving a referral, the co-ordinator or her assistant visits the family, tells them about the nature of Scope and what it can offer and invites the mother to attend a local group with her pre-school children. If the mother accepts the invitation, she is contacted by the group's convenor who offers to accompany her to the group and introduce her to other members. In this way, Scope tries to ensure that new parents are made to feel welcome. In 1979/80, 66 per cent of the families visited joined the groups. The proportion for the previous two years was 52 per cent and 46 per cent respectively. About one-fifth of those who did not join the groups were visited at home by members of Scope and wherever necessary this home visiting was continued, sometimes for long periods of time.

The management committee   Perhaps one of the more unusual features of Scope's organisation (which may in itself prove a model for other care-giving agencies) lies in the structure of its management committee. This is composed of representatives from the local health, education and social services together with representatives from each of the thirteen neighbourhood groups. The managment committee carries out the central administration of Scope and determines its policy. The full-time co-ordinator and her part-time assistant are employed by the committee and are accountable to it. This management structure gives the neighbourhood groups and the different statutory and voluntary services an unusual opportunity to work together. The statutory services have a source of information about families' ideas, complaints and appreciation of their work. For their part, the families have access to information and advice on the various statutory services in their neighbourhoods.

The co-ordinators and group convenors   The SSRC report of this scheme observes the unusual degree of trust and collaboration between Scope and the statutory services. Their research suggests that this owes much to the emphasis placed on the preparation and continuous support of the group convenors and the project co-ordinators.   Group convenors undertake a training course before they take responsibility for a Scope group. The course is run by the co-ordinator and consists of ten sessions over a ten-week period.   After this, group convenors all receive support in their work through regular meetings with a community psychiatrist and senior social worker. They also meet with the co-ordinator for regular training sessions. For their part, the co-ordinator and assistant co-ordinator have access to professional supervision from a senior social worker.

By these methods, Scope has gradually built up in each of their groups' neighbourhoods a small number of skilled volunteer family workers. They are available for visiting families with problems as well as for running groups. The training of these convenors helps them identify the limitations of their own skills and the importance of identifying the point at which they should call in extra help from the co-ordinator. She in turn can quickly call upon professional assistance through her close links on the management committee with the health, social and educational services in Southampton.   The SSRC research emphasises the importance of this role definition in achieving the co-operation of the statutory services.   Scope does not attempt to substitute for the statutory services but offers a complementary type of support. '. . . the principles are clear, the philosophy is right and there is a boundary between what they can do and what social workers can do.'

Arbour, Liverpool[20]

Although the number of births to girls aged 16 years or less has decreased slightly since the early 1970s, the health problems of these babies and their mothers continue to be matters for concern. With other teenage pregnancies their perinatal and infant mortality rates are higher than that of the total population (McAnarney, E.R. 1978; OPCS 1983d).   Studies have shown that young teenage mothers often attend antenatal and child health clinics infrequently, late or not at all (National Council for One Parent Families 1979).   This pattern of low service contact is also found in other sectors of care which may be equally important to the health and wellbeing of the young mother and her infant — for instance, education and social services.   Loss of schooling at a time when the mother should be acquiring the necessary qualifications to secure later employment may result in the new baby being born into a home with a predetermined level of poverty due to low earning capacity.

In Liverpool the health, educational and social needs of this small but vulnerable group have become the focus for a special collaborative scheme known initially as the Pregnant Schoolgirls Project.   In 1980 it was renamed the Arbour Project.   Its origins can be traced back to 1977 when an inter-departmental working party was established to examine the local provision of pregnancy counselling services in the city for children under sixteen.   The formation of this group was prompted by the recommendations of the Lane Committee on the working of the Abortion Act (Lane 1974).   Included in the working party were representatives from the education, health and social services, as well as the voluntary organisation known as the Liverpool Personal Social Services Society.

It was estimated that at the time at least one hundred and fifty schoolgirls in Liverpool became pregnant every year.   Although approximately half of these had abortions, the remaining seventy or so continued with their pregnancies.   The education department were concerned that they knew of only about thirty pregnancies a year in the 11—16 age group.   Clearly, there was a need to co-ordinate the services for all these girls, whether they had abortions or not.   There was also a need to provide friendly and accessible services which encouraged those who decided to have their babies to continue with their education and obtain the maximum use of antenatal care.

The Pregnant Schoolgirl Project was set up in 1978 to try and meet these needs.   Contributions came from many quarters.   The senior social workers at the Young Peoples Advisory Service of the Liverpool Personal Services Society see every girl referred to the project for immediate counselling and information. This is also available for her boyfriend and family. In this way it is hoped that the parents-to-be can decide which course their pregnancies should take, having regard to all the options. The social workers also provide a weekly group counselling session for girls in the project. In 1981 the Liverpool Personal Services Society employed a part-time nursery nurse to work with Arbour. Among other things she has established a toy library and a mother-and-toddler group. Both these activities have helped to extend the project's services to girls who are no longer of school age.

For those who decide to continue with their pregnancy, the education department provides various ways of completing their education: in their own school, at home or in a special class for schoolgirl mothers. A home teacher has been seconded, full time, to run this class. It has been housed in a variety of places including a health clinic and a disused school. The class is now in more permanent premises and provides places for 12 girls at any one time.

The health authority has appointed a part-time maternity and child health visitor with a special responsibility for the project. Her work is to complement, rather than replace, the care which the girls receive from their own midwives and health visitors. As well as being a health advisor to the pregnant schoolgirls, the health visitor works closely with the rest of the project team. On one afternoon every week she runs a health education session. This is informal and covers subjects chosen to cover the needs and interests of the group. Girls are welcomed to the session from the moment they make contact with the project — whether they are continuing their education in school, in the special class or at home. They are encouraged to continue with their weekly meetings after their baby is born. The health visitor emphasised the important contribution which these postnatal mothers make to the rest of the group by sharing their own experiences of pregnancy and childbirth.

The matrons of the social service department's day nurseries provide mothercraft sessions. This link between the project and the day nursery was established at the start of the project so that mothers could place their new babies in a day nursery while they went out to work or continued schooling.

In 1980 the project acquired a grant of £10,000 per annum for five years from the health authority's Joint Finance budget. This injection of funds has allowed them to employ a part-time project co-ordinator to work with the project team. One of her main tasks has been to improve referral procedures so that an increasing proportion of pregnant schoolgirls in Liverpool are made aware of the project's services and put in touch with them.

In doing this she has worked closely with the Principal Education Welfare Officer and many other individuals in the various statutory and voluntary services in Liverpool.

But to return to the health service's part in Arbour. Since the start of the project, liaison with midwives in the antenatal clinics has ensured that, with mothers' permission, their names and addresses are passed to the project as soon as they book for antenatal care. The clinic midwives tell the project health visitor of any significant difficulties during the girls' pregnancies. They also contact her if they lose touch with a mother. Health visitor liaison posts have now been established in every maternity hospital booking clinic in the city. These health visitors also work closely with the project.

Predictions from previous research suggest that this group of schoolgirl mothers would be poor attenders at clinics and health education sessions. Yet they have all been to virtually everything to which the health service and project have invited them. It is *over*-attendance rather than under-attendance which is beginning to stretch the limited resources of this small project. Many of the girls continue attending the health education sessions for several months after their baby is born. For some their contact with the project is even longer. A girl who dropped out of college after the birth of her baby returned for support when her baby was fourteen months old. Another of the mothers who had left school came back and attended the group regularly during her second pregnancy.

There may be various interpretations of this apparent success story. The numbers of mothers who have been through the project are small, representing less than half the pregnant school-girls in Liverpool. The girls are a self-selected group and may not be representative of all pregnant schoolgirls. I would risk a more positive, if tentative, interpretation. Quite simply, the experience of Arbour suggests that the so called 'hard-to-reach', high-risk groups in pregnancy may become easy to reach when services are modified adequately to meet their needs. One aspect of these modifications is probably the amount of personal attention which each of the teenage mothers receives from the project team, and especially from the health visitor. Another is the way all the different aspects of pregnancy care for health are combined together into the single service of Arbour.

Family Start, Oldham[21]

Family Start aims to meet the needs of parents and infants living on Sholver, a modern yet decaying council estate isolated on the northern edge of Oldham; in this difficult environment it attempts to promote health through good parenting and family relationships.

Funding and staff   Family Start was initiated by the local Family Service Unit (part of a national voluntary organisation) in 1978 with an urban aid grant of some £13,000 per year for five years. Its team consists of a health visitor, fieldwork teacher (the project co-ordinator), a qualified social worker seconded by the social services department, someone trained in counselling and group work, and two part-time secretaries.   The overall responsibility for the project lies with the Family Service Unit organiser to whom the project co-ordinator is accountable.

Preparatory work   The preparatory phase of Family Start was intended to last only three months but took nine to complete. The team emphasised the necessity of this lead-in time to get to know the community and statutory services working on the estate.   They listened and talked with pregnant mothers and families with young babies and gradually built up a picture of people's lives, their types of problem and the support and care they wanted.   They also worked to gain the trust of the health professionals providing these families with antenatal and child health services.

Key features: their approach   From the start of the project the team have allowed themselves to experiment with new ways of working, responding with their pooled resources and skills to the needs which they and the families identify.   The co-ordinator compared her Family Start experience with her previous work as a nursing officer in a health authority:

> There I was concerned, day in, day out, with maintaining and monitoring more of the same.   There wasn't the time or the opportunity to try even a little of something different.   I was certainly never exposed to so many ideas about different ways of working.

After some months the team formulated their approach.   Whenever possible their work would be preventive; they would aim to reach *all* mothers with a first or second pregnancy in the early months; they would try to avoid parents' dependency on their services; they would evaluate their progress.

Contacting parents   At the outset, the GPs' weekly antenatal clinic and the health visitors' and midwives' routine home visits were used for distributing information about the project.   With parents' permission, community nurses passed their addresses to Family Start.   These methods of contact were not entirely satisfactory as not all parents attended the clinic and the health visitors' and midwives' visits usually occurred late in pregnancy.

So ways are being found to contact parents through the hospital antenatal clinics.

It was estimated that in one year between 90 to 100 women living within the project area would have a first or second baby (the only ones the project catered for). In the first year of the project approximately 70 pregnant women were identified by the procedures outlined above. Only 3 of these were not interviewed.

Once names and addresses of new parents are obtained, the co-ordinator writes to ask if one of the team may visit. With consent, a team member, using a structured questionnaire, systematically reviews with each mother her housing and financial situation, her education and her recollections about her own childhood experiences. She is asked about this pregnancy and birth: for instance, the changes the new baby will create in the family, the details of her diet and her plans for having future children. Her knowledge of the various maternity and child health services is also explored. At this interview parents may identify areas of possible difficulty, and the interviewer can suggest ways in which Family Start may be able to help; for instance, information about welfare rights, maternity benefits and housing. A personal counselling service is offered for emotional and family problems. Problems specifically concerned with the mother's or baby's health can be assessed by the team member who is a health visitor and referred to the appropriate part of the health service.

Parents' contracts   When parents have identified problem areas and know the services which the project provides, the decision to take them up rests with the parents. If they decide to go ahead they make a contract with Family Start for specific difficulties to be worked on in defined ways over a set period of time.

Within a month after the birth, Family Start contacts the parents again to find out how they are coping. They assess if there are any changes in the parents' home or family situation, and, if required, new contracts are negotiated for specific problems with which assistance is requested.

Family Start have now opened a drop-in centre for parents on the estate, and have initiated an ambitious research programme to evaluate their work.

In conclusion

The efficiency and effectiveness of the community resources for health may be improved if the statutory and voluntary services which normally work separately for the wellbeing of families find ways of working together. Everything possible should be done to reduce the barriers which fracture rather than unite our family services. The schemes described in this chapter suggest a few of the many ways in which this might be done in neighbourhoods, health authorities and general practices.

The process of forming partnerships usually results in changes both for the individuals and the organisations involved. In the course of this study it has become apparent that there are probably several ingredients necessary for coping with the uncertainties and questioning that will almost inevitably result: plenty of preparation, training and support for the individuals involved together with the necessary financial and administrative backing from their organisations. In addition, there is the dimension of time. It appears that building trusting relationships between people and organisations who normally work apart may take years.

Finally it must be emphasised that the approaches to promoting inter-agency collaboration described in this chapter may have little impact if they are not paralleled by a greater degree of co-ordination between central government departments concerned with the family. These approaches are also threatened by recent cuts in public expenditure, which are likely to undermine the development of greater inter-agency collaboration as they reduce the financial, professional and organisational commitment for such ventures.

Notes

1 The term 'agency' covers the statutory and voluntary organisations concerned with care for health at the local level. These include health authorities, family practitioner committees and community health councils and their various services; also local authority departments concerned with policy issues and services which may affect parent and child health. Also included are voluntary organisations and their intermediary bodies, for instance councils of voluntary service.

2 Dr J. Williamson, 91 Dodworth Road, Barnsley, South Yorkshire S70 6HB.

3 Dr C. Smith, Health Centre, Thatcham, Berks.

4 Health authorities in Birmingham, Coventry, Ealing and Hillingdon have also 'detached' their health visitors from general practitioners.

5 This decrease in numbers was due to the redeployment of staff. Overall, there was no decrease in the numbers of community nurses covering Barnsley.

6 District Co-ordinator of Voluntary Services, Charing Cross Hospital, Fulham Palace Road, London W6 8RF.

7 Dr Tom Heller, 246 Darnell Road, Darnell, Sheffield.

8 Judith Elkan, Lisson Grove Health Centre Project, Department of Child Psychiatry, Paddington Green Children's Hospital, Paddington Green, London W2 1LQ.

9 Gwen Hiskins HV, 34 Barrow Point Avenue, Pinner, Middlesex.

10 The Co-ordinator, Newpin, Sutherland House, Sutherland Square, Walworth Road, London SE17.

11 It should be noted that the recommended exclusion of lay members from professional discussions, such as perinatal audits, has been criticised by

some of the main consumer groups involved in maternity care. To quote the Maternity Alliance, 'Only when the tokenism of 'lay membership' is replaced by an acceptance of the consumer as *Specialist* in the use of services will we find a significant change in antenatal practice' (Maternity Action 1982, no 7).

12 Antenatal Health Project, NCVO, 26 Bedford Square, London WC1B 3HU.
13 Good Practices in Maternity Services Project (Janet Finucane), Manchester CHC, 1 St Anne's Churchyard, Manchester 2.
14 Good Practices in Maternity Services Project (Harry Trent), Southern Sheffield CHC, Westfield House, 81 Division Street, Sheffield S1 4HT.
15 Good Practices in Maternity Services Project (John Bradwell), Cleveland CVS, 49 Princes Road, Middlesbrough, South Tees.
16 Martin Bradley, Liverpool Institute of Higher Education, Stand Park Road, Liverpool L16 9JD.
17 Sue Dowling, Canynge Hall, Whiteladies Road, Bristol BS8 2PR.
18 Geoff Poulton, Department of Sociology and Social Administration, University of Southampton SO9 5NH.
19 Lin Poulton, The Firs, West End, Southampton.
20 The Co-ordinator, Arbour Project, 161A Dakfield Road, Liverpool 4.
21 The Co-ordinator, Family Start, Family Service Unit, 3/5 Hamilton Street, Oldham OL4 1DA.

10 Parents and children as active participants in health care

'People have the right and the duty to participate individually and collectively in the planning and implementation of their health care. Consequently, community involvement in shaping its own health and socioeconomic future, including mass involvement of women, men and youth, is a key factor in the strategy.'

(World Health Organisation. *Global Strategy for Health for All by the Year 2000*. Para II. 9(3). 1981)

The emphasis throughout this book has been on the *providers* of preventive health care in pregnancy and early childhood: the NHS, local authority services and the voluntary sector. Yet many of the schemes described suggest the importance of liberating ourselves from straight-jacket thinking about 'active' providers and 'passive' receivers of care. In the course of this study, it has been apparent that many parents and children want greater involvement in their health care.

There is a danger, however, that for health professionals, consumer involvement in disease prevention and health promotion will be limited to a modification of personal habits like smoking, drinking, diet and attendance at relevant clinics. Consumerism in health may also be seen as a development which will cause little disturbance to the way professionals work or to the structure and power relationships within the NHS. The experience of this study suggests otherwise. People are asking for a larger share in information and influence in many areas which may affect their health: in the way in which their health services are planned and organised and the control of environmental and social health hazards in their districts. There are examples from this study where health workers have welcomed the contributions of lay persons and have found ways to work collaboratively. It must be stressed however, that parents who have tried to influence local health issues have more often reported insuperable difficulties due to the negative attitudes of professionals, problems in obtaining relevant information and lack of power compared with the professionals who plan and run the health services.

Despite the professional and political opposition which it may receive, everything I learned from this study suggests that consumerism, with its demands for greater participation in health and health care, is likely to continue to increase. Schemes in which parents and children are actively contributing to the design and running of their own local health care suggest the energy, ideas and resources which may be unlocked by this type of process. Indeed, as the study has progressed I have gradually realised that one reason for the health service's difficulty in reaching certain families with preventive health care may be our failure to recognise that in every consumer there is a potential provider.

It has not been possible to mention all the schemes which illustrate the way in which parents and young children are trying to have a direct influence on issues concerning their health and health services. Some are described in previous chapters — for instance the work of certain mutual-aid health groups in attempting to improve the training of health professionals and the design of services. In this chapter I will confine myself to three main areas of consumerism in health — namely Community Health Councils, patient participation groups in general practice, and neighbourhood health projects.

Community Health Councils

CHCs are statutory bodies which exist in every district to represent the views and interests of the public to their health authority. Members are appointed by local authorities, the regional health authority and voluntary organisations. It should be noted that CHCs have no executive power in health service decisions or management: they act as advisors, sources of information and, where necessary, as pressure groups for the users of health services.

Many CHCs have outlined ways in which they are trying to improve the access and availability of maternity and preventive child health services for families. Some of them pointed to changes in services such as clinics which seemed to be a direct result of their action. However, most were less certain of their impact, and were aware of their limited power by comparison with professionals in the health service. The following summary indicates the main type of activities reported by CHCs.

Information to assist parents in their choice of health care

With information collected from health authorities and their own investigations, some CHCs give parents detailed advice about the availability and characteristics of the different maternity and child health services in their district. They may advise parents on which clinics have play facilities for children and which GPs are sympathetic to women wanting home births, and CHCs (like Oxford and Ealing) have published this information in pamphlets.

Influencing planning and operation of NHS services

— CHCs are available for people's complaints about the antenatal and child health services: problems of long waiting times, transport and child care when attending clinics are often mentioned. Where appropriate these complaints are passed on to the health authority.

— Some CHCs arrange clinics visits regularly to talk to staff and parents. In Coventry[1] these visits led the CHC to make a series of recommendations for greater comfort and more convenient timing. Many of these recommendations have been implemented by the health authority.

— Surveys have been carried out to provide information about the consumers' perspective of the preventive antenatal and child health services and how they can be improved. (See for instance Kensington, Chelsea and Westminster (South) CHC 1980; Kidderminster CHC 1978; Central Birmingham CHC 1981.) CHCs sometimes mentioned problems in carrying out such surveys: difficulties in obtaining the necessary research advice and assistance, in obtaining permission from certain health professionals to carry out the studies, problems of finance, and reluctance by the health authority to respond to the council's findings. (For a review of CHC surveys of antenatal care, see Garcia, J. 1981.)

— CHCs are asked to give their views on health authority plans for maternity and child health services. Some are represented on district planning teams which advise the district management team on the planning and operation of these services. (See p. 137.)

— A few CHCs have helped initiate special community health projects to contribute to local preventive maternity care — see for instance City and Hackney CHC[2], p. 38.

Health education: St Thomas's Children's Health Club

CHCs occasionally described their involvement in health education projects to develop the public's knowledge of preventive maternity and child health issues: Cardiff CHC[3] helped a women's group in Adamstown, an inner city neighbourhood, to establish a Women and Health Course. Coventry CHC, concerned about low take-up of immunisation, asked the health authority to produce map posters, indicating the districts of the city in which childhood immunisation rates were particularly low, to inform the public.
An unusual and surprisingly popular health education scheme is

the Children's Health Club, set up with local children by St Thomas's Community Health Council.[4] The club meets regularly in the council's offices. Members come from the nearby flats and estate and are from many different ethnic and social backgrounds.

The essence of the club's philosophy is that health issues are fun and that young children can enthusiastically design and take responsibility in neighbourhood health programmes and be effective teachers. With the support of a few adults, members have learned to run the club, plan activities and acquire information about health. Since 1978, a particular feature of the club has been a programme in which members teach other children about dental health care (Plamping, D. *et al.* 1980). They visit schools, hospitals, youth clubs, GPs' surgeries and playgrounds. Involved adults confirm that the children's knowledge of dental care has increased considerably, as well as their self-confidence. Parents, teachers and others at the CHC commented on the surprising level of responsibility which children have assumed and fulfilled. For a further description of this project, see Smith, R. 1981.

Patient participation in general practice

In the last decade a form of consumer representation in health care has evolved called Patient Participation Groups in General Practice (Pritchard, P. 1981). Inevitably, such groups tend to develop only in practices where the GPs make them welcome. At the beginning of 1983, it was estimated that there were some forty groups throughout England, Scotland and Wales. In 1978 a National Association[5] for these groups was formed to support and promote their further development.[6]

Most participation groups are composed of patient members of the general practice who wish to influence and be involved in the planning and nature of the health service. Groups usually have regular meetings, often with the practice staff. Such an approach:

> challenges the adequacy and appropriateness of a profession always assuming that it knows what is best for the community it serves . . . it recognises the very positive contribution that can and should be made to community health care by all those who live in it.
> (Paine, T. 1983)

A survey of these groups in 1981 indicated that they have helped to bring about the appointment of women partners, improvements in surgery waiting areas, the introduction of a crèche in well-baby clinics and changed visiting arrangements in a local children's ward (Paine, T. 1983).

A health education scheme in Aberdare

A project from Aberdare,[7] South Wales, shows how patient participation groups can identify local needs and devise new approaches to meet them. The Aberdare patients committee were concerned that many local parents were doubtful about immunisation for their babies. Health professionals tended to emphasise the advantages yet, through the media, parents had learned about dangers, such as brain damage.

The committee reacted with a special health education programme. They designed it to reach as many parents as possible, particularly those who were unlikely to come to public health education meetings held at the health centre. With the assistance of their health authority, they planned and made their own video film. A local and well-known health visitor and a paediatrician answered questions about immunisation from a group of parents at the health centre. The film — which had already attracted considerable local attention — was then taken to homes on nearby estates, where a mother acted as host and invited other parents from the area. Members of the committee also led a follow-up discussion (for further details of the patients' committee, see Wilson, A. 1977).

Neighbourhood health projects

CHCs and Patient Participation Groups are examples of consumer groups which have developed within the framework of the NHS organisation. In contrast, neighbourhood health projects are independent of the health service and are based in local communities. Though still relatively few in number, this type of project is of special interest because of the use of the community development approach to health promotion, which has been successfully employed in community health programmes in developing countries for many years (Newell, K. 1975). In this country, however, such ways of working have only recently evolved as possible solutions to the inequalities in health experienced by the poorest sections of society (Kings Fund Centre 1980; Smith, C. 1982). The following are characteristics which tend to typify projects using this approach:

— They are neighbourhood-based and emphasise the relationship between people's health and the local social, economic and environmental factors which may affect it. E.g. unemployment, poor housing, dangerous roads, inaccessible health services.

— They assist people to organise themselves to take confident responsibility in determining their own health needs and ways of meeting them.

— The starting-point of these programmes are worries and concerns of local people — health needs of mothers and young children as perceived by the community rather than by the health professionals who serve it. Thornhill Neighbourhood Project[8] has carried out an investigation of antenatal care in their area based on the experience of local women. This has involved a questionnaire-based survey and a series of group meetings held on local estates so that women can further develop their ideas about the services they want (Thornhill Neighbourhood Project 1982).

— Self-help groups and voluntary schemes may be established to challenge the power of professionals and help demystify their expertise. 'Health in Homerton'[9] (a community project based on a Hackney housing estate) has worked with pregnant women to make their visits to the antenatal clinic in the health centre more enjoyable. They have set up a support group for pregnant women which meets weekly in one of their homes (Robinson, J. and Rosenthal, H. 1981).

— Projects are usually staffed by community workers rather than health professionals.

The following descriptions of three neighbourhood projects only give a flavour of this type of work, but, though they have not been formally evaluated, they suggest the potential of this approach to preventive health care in impoverished urban neighbourhoods. These examples all come from London, but neighbourhood health projects are now developing in other towns. In 1983 the National Council for Voluntary Organisations established a unit to disseminate information and assist new ones to develop.[10]

The Peckham Health Project

This project[11] is based in a flat on an estate in south London, and was initiated by the Pitt Street Settlement. The main worker in the project is a community worker, supported by a GP from a nearby health centre and a planning group of local people. A health group has been established as part of the project; it is open to anyone but is composed mainly of women with young children from the estate. They meet regularly and undertake a variety of activities: organising public meetings on various health topics, working with the King's District Health Campaign to investigate the effects of cuts to their health services and forming special-interest groups e.g. on child health, stopping smoking, cystitis and thrush.

An important part of the project's work is to demystify health information and make it available to local people. Members of the special-interest groups have written their own health education pamphlets on coping with childhood illnesses, breast-feeding, parental depression, cystitis and thrush:

> . . . finding out information, discussing it amongst a group of people and understanding it enough to put it in language that is generally understood is an achievement in itself. Tackling complicated medical information which one would once have thought to be the territory of doctors in an even greater accomplishment . . . Groups have found this very rewarding. Secondly, this is a way that people are able to pass on information they have picked up . . . it would become pointless and esoteric if all we were doing was creating a few more people who had knowledge that they were unable or unwilling to share.
>
> (Peckham Health Project 1979)

Another objective of the project is to increase people's confidence to control their own health and the factors which influence it. The 'smoke stop' group also tried to prevent local shops from selling cigarettes to children under-age, and displayed anti-smoking information at community events. Women in the health group learned to tackle their anxieties when confronting doctors and other health professionals by role-playing 'doctors and patients' and by making a video film about doctor/patient communication. The health group have used this video film for medical students and GP trainees to understand consultations from the patients' point of view. (For a further account of this neighbourhood project see Peckham Health Project Report 1979.)

The Bermondsey Lamp Post

> The area where we live is south of the river between Tower Bridge and London Bridge . . . The riverside stagnates; local industries and shops close, and improving the quality of life for adult or child is a policy but not an active priority. Our local area social services office is infamous for its under-manning, its inner disputes and a recent lengthy strike. Our surgeries are increasingly locked up, our chemists disappear, and we scramble like ants around the base of the mammoth tower block of our local hospital, seeking entry with the qualifications of being a local resident, to find that we have been relegated to a place in the queue along with the rest of south-east England . . . There is a strong feeling that we are serviced from without; few in health or social work or teaching actually live here, but each day we are serviced by an influx of professionals who feel that they know best for our own good. There is a definite feeling of 'them' and 'us', a legacy of years of misapplied professionalism . . .
>
> (Parent and resident of Bermondsey Street, London S.W.1)

The starting-point of the Bermondsey Lamp Post project[12] in 1972 was the concern of local parents, children and a few teachers about the impoverished educational and play provision in a small inner city neighbourhood south of the Thames. A teacher who lived in the area acted initially as an unpaid community worker. Derelict land was opened up for play areas and holiday play schemes were organised. Later, a Free School, known as the Bermondsey Lamp Post, was established by the community worker and local people to provide education for a maximum of thirty children from the neighbourhood.

Two doctors came to live in the area: a registrar in paediatrics from the nearby teaching hospital and a clinical medical officer who worked at the child health clinic and in the primary schools of the area. Living in the same area as the families with whom they worked they could see the mismatches of the services provided and families' needs, and were able to feed this information back into the health service. Their identity as next-door neighbours rather than as professionals often gave them the necessary accepta-ability to reach vulnerable families who were reluctant to contact statutory services. Like the other workers in the project, they became intimately involved in a wide range of children's activities, including schooling, recreation, holidays and care of animals, thus providing many opportunities for children, parents and health workers to share their information. Health education became an agenda-less and continuing process.

Encouraging families to use the local hospitals and clinics was an important aspect of the project's work. This was achieved in ways requiring considerable organisation and support to ensure that children were not rebuffed by busy professionals. When Polly the dog was sick, or a pigeon found dying in the road, the children went to the casualty department to ask for advice and materials for their resuscitation; when engaged in school projects on teeth and bones, they were directed to a friendly person in the dental school and the department of surgery for information. As the children got to know some professionals within the hospital as friends, it was hoped that they would learn to be at home in its rather large and impersonal buildings. They might also gain some skills necessary for approaching professionals directly for help.

As well as these activities, local families made their own con-tribution to the available resources for health in the area. At the time of writing, they have raised much of the funding necessary for a family centre for local parents, young children and old age pensioners. Like the Peckham Health Project, parents have become involved in teaching medical students, hoping that this will alert them to the health problems of the neighbourhood. Mutual aid has also been a feature of the project's work: individuals who have experienced abortion or a particular illness have acted as counsellors for others in similar situations; mothers who have breast-fed their babies encourage and support others to do the same. Parents connected with the project have also gained the acceptance of the staff in their hospital antenatal clinic, and have been allowed to set up a crèche that provides play and refreshments. The majority of women who run it had babies in the hospital, and can provide an informal source of information to local expectant mothers.

Early in 1980, a parallel organisation to the Bermondsey Lamp Post was formed, known as the Bermondsey Street Community Association. This is composed of neighbourhood residents and the accent of the group is on improving the polluted and noisy inner city environment and providing family facilities. Much of their work is therefore directly relevant to health promotion. Aware that road traffic accidents are a major cause of childhood death and injury, the association has had a safety barrier erected outside a local estate to prevent children from running into the road; mothers on an estate surrounded by heavy traffic routes were concerned about the dangers of lead pollution. Through the community association they have brought this to the attention of their Environmental Health Officer who has monitored the lead levels in the streets. Parents in the association have also alerted this officer to the pollution and nuisance caused by local firms burning noxious chemical waste, and the excessive noise caused by the air-cooling system of a nearby tower block. In both these cases action has been taken to eliminate the problems.

Stockwell Health Project and the Mawbey Brough Health Centre

Mawbey Brough is a rundown inner city area where the old housing stock — mainly council-owned — is being demolished. A new health centre has been proposed in the redevelopment plan for the area. St Thomas' CHC were concerned about the lack of community consultation and joined with the Stockwell and Vauxhall Neighbourhood Council to collect residents' views on how they would like to see their new health centre develop. Out of this venture has grown the Stockwell Health Project[13], made up of local people wanting to organise around health issues — as in the previously described Peckham Project. Though closely related to the Community Health Council and Neighbourhood Council, the project considers itself independent of them. A grant from the King Edward VII Hospital Fund has enabled the health project to employ a community health worker.

The initial working group, set up by the CHC and Neighbourhood Council, identified about twenty community groups which expressed interest in the health centre: tenants' associations, playgroups, children's clubs, mother-and-toddler groups, pensioners' groups and an art centre. Most of these were visited, as were many individuals at home, to get their ideas for the proposed centre. Many of them wanted to be involved and felt they had something to give, yet were convinced they were powerless to persuade health professionals that their ideas were worth considering.

Within a year the working group published a report: 'Mawbey Brough — A Health Centre for the Community?' This presented their findings and suggested ways in which the health centre plans could incorporate the community's wishes:

> The collective experience of these community groups has shown what the community can achieve for itself. However, in a deprived area such as Stockwell, these achievements have to be supported, especially as they unearth issues of greater concern for the community, notably health. These can only be tackled if sympathetic and adequate support is available. The facilities, resources and people centred in the new health centre could be an opportunity to provide that support in an exciting and imaginative way so that the people of Stockwell are encouraged to play a very real part in assuming responsibility for their own health.

Perhaps one of the most important recommendations of the report was that there should be direct community involvement in the managing body of the health centre.

The working group and then the Stockwell Health Project had a long and painful struggle to achieve recognition of their ideas and suggestions by their health authority. They reported that replies to their letters were slow — if they came at all. There were difficulties in finding the appropriate person in the health authority to give them the information they needed. Problems arose when they tried to ascertain the authority's timetable for the centre's planning — which decisions would be made by whom and when. In presenting their case in an acceptable way to the various officers and committees of the health authority, the group had to prepare reports and submit alternative architectural plans. The costs of these had to be found from a variety of sources including the Community Health Council.

Despite these difficulties Stockwell Health Project, with help from a sympathetic district community physician, eventually engaged the district management team in discussion. Their requests for representation on the health authority's project group responsible for planning the health centre initially appeared to be ignored. Later, after prolonged and insistent negotiations, the original project group was disbanded and a new one established to advise the district management team on the planning of the health centre.

The membership of this newly constituted group consists of five representatives of the district health authority and up to six members of the community from the Stockwell Health Project. Other community representatives may be invited to meetings to discuss items relevant to them — for instance, services for families in pregnancy and early childhood. The post of chairman and secretary rotate at three-monthly intervals, with a community representative holding one post and a health authority representative the other. Part of the function of this new project group has been to suggest an acceptable procedure by which community representatives will be involved in the health centre's policy-making and also in the evaluation of the centre's services.

This venture in shared professional and public involvement in neighbourhood health service planning is certainly unusual and may be unique. It is important that it is carefully monitored to chart its difficulties and advantages and to see whether it results in the burgeoning of local resources and interest in health which, at its outset, it promises.

In conclusion

The position of the consumer in matters of health and health services has, until recently, been one of relative powerlessness. It appears that in maternity and pre-school health care, as well as health care in general, things are gradually changing. In the future, the development of collaboration between the users and providers of health services, though likely to be an uneasy process, may add new dimensions of resources, skills and approaches to health promotion in the community. It seems important that those working in the NHS recognise these positive aspects of consumerism in health care and find ways in which parents and children can be drawn further into the planning and organisation of their health services: by greater involvement in health service planning groups, maternity services liaison committees, the training of health professionals and through more informal methods of consultation and collaboration at the neighbourhood level.

However, it must be appreciated that the increase of consumer interest in health care, which enables relatively powerless groups to become powerful, may appear threatening to many professionals. They will be asked to establish new types of relationships with the users of services in which participation means far more than token consultation and discussion. It is unlikely that such a major shift in practice can occur without considerable attention to the training and support of the health professionals concerned. Training establishments and health authorities should consider how they can provide health workers with opportunities to learn about the different types of consumer participation in health care which are developing. They should also teach about their value and the way in which they can work with them.

Finally, as with all the new developments described in this book, there is a need to chart the progress in consumer participation in health care and study its impact. It will be important to evaluate how these innovations influence attitudes and knowledge about health and illness, the way in which parents and children relate to the health services, and their experience of illness.

Notes

1   Coventry CHC, Room 222, Broadgate House, Broadgate, Coventry CB1 1NG.
2   City and Hackney CHC, 210 Kingsland Road, London E2 8EB.
3   Cardiff CHC, 15 St David's House, Wood Street, Cardiff.
4   St Thomas' CHC, 2 Cleaver Road, London SE11.
5   National Association for Patient Participation, c/o Hazelbank, Peaslake, Guildford, Surrey GU5 9RJ.
6   In 1983 the Royal College of General Practitioners set up a Patient's Liaison Group through which patients will have the opportunity to tell the College their views on various aspects of general practice.
7   Patients Committee, The Health Centre, High Street, Aberdare, Mid Glamorgan.
8   Thornhill Neighbourhood Project, Orkney House, 199 Caledonian Road, London N1.
9   'Health in Homerton', c/o City and Hackney CHC, 210 Kingsland Road, London E2 8EB.
10 NCVO, Community Health Initiatives Resource Unit, 26 Bedford Square, London WC1B 3HU.
11 Peckham Health Project, c/o Pitt Street Settlement, 191 East Surrey Grove, Peckham, London SE15 5PP.
12 Lois Acton, 96 Grosvenor Terrace, London SE5.
13 Stockwell Health Project, c/o Stockwell and Vauxhall Neighbourhood Council, 157 South Lambert Road, London SW8.

11 An overview

In recent years a succession of major reports have encouraged new
and imaginative approaches to the delivery of preventive health
care in the community. The names of Court (1976), Short (1980),
Merrison (1979), Black (1980) and Acheson (1981) are just a few
of those associated with these recommendations. This book has
mapped out the variety of ways in which these policy ideals are
beginning to be translated into practice in the maternity and child
health services in different parts of England and Wales. It is based
on a study which is primarily descriptive and which has considered
the delivery of preventive health care at all levels (primary, secondary and tertiary), in a variety of situations — not just antenatal
and child health clinics.

In previous chapters, I have drawn conclusions from the particular schemes described. Now I move away from the particular, and
identify some of the main issues which emerge from the study as a
whole. The most impressive of these must be that with adequate
resources, motivation and imagination, our preventive maternity
and pre-school services for health could be transformed into ones
which are attractive and readily available for modern families. The
success of many of the projects described in this book puts the lie
to the belief that certain groups of parents and young children,
especially those most economically and socially disadvantaged, are
particularly difficult, perhaps even impossible, to reach with
preventive health care. Where attention is given to parents' life
styles and needs, and services are modified and redesigned, it
appears that most families *can* be contacted, and often with
surprising ease.

The manner in which these schemes have evolved emphasises
the essential role of *creativity* in the planning process for preventive
health: experimenting with imaginative and different ways of
delivering care, moving into new territories of skills, exploring
previously untested partnerships with agencies and individuals
working outside the NHS. If new ways are to be found to meet
the health needs created by the rapid changes in the population's
economic, social and demographic characteristics such creativity
seems essential. It is clear from this study that there is no shortage
of it within the NHS, or in the other services concerned with
health.

However it appears that in the NHS there is some reluctance to
recognise, promote and utilise this creativity for change. In part

this may be due to the increasing emphasis on scientific management: of measuring, monitoring and evaluating the efficiency of
that which already exists and is done. Of course, these activities
are important. But we would do well to recall Bruner's reminder
of the metaphor of the left and right hand and its relevance to the
growth of knowledge (Bruner, J. 1973). The right is the hand of
taught reason and precision. The left is the dreamer, sometimes
awkward, but with the daring to project into the unknown and
uncertain. In different ways *both* hands are essential. The function
of one without the other is much reduced.

It could be argued, however, that at times of uncertainty —
such as the recent restructuring of the NHS and the swingeing cuts
to health authority and local authority budgets — resistance to
anything new is a necessary prerequisite for survival. A major
function of management must be that of keeping going and of
working strictly within the framework of what exists and is already
known. If new developments are needed — as they are now —
they will have to be most energetically promoted.

In the promotion of innovation, it should be noted that in this
study much of the creativity for improved delivery of health care
came from fieldworkers who are close to the needs of families and
distant from the responsibilities of managing large organisations.
This observation is reminiscent of other studies which have pointed
to the importance of the 'bottom up' approach to change in
services (see, for instance, Towell, D. and Harries, C. 1979). The
ideas and experience of people who are relatively junior in the
hierarchy of the NHS structure need to reach their more senior
managers and be incorporated into the planning of health care. It
seems that within the NHS these links are not always made. The
suggestion of development agencies for the NHS (Hunter, D. 1983),
deserves serious consideration. They may provide one way of
overcoming these difficulties and stimulating innovation in health
service organisation and delivery. Such an agency would have a
different approach from the experimental Management Advisory
Services which appear to function as an inspectorate, focusing on
monitoring and standard-setting (Ham, C. and McMahon, L. 1982).
A development agency:

> would make innovation less of a hit and miss activity . . . It
> would act locally with those who make decisions and provide
> the services, encouraging them to become agents for change.
> The agency would be a catalyst operating on a consultancy basis
> offering help and support to service providers. Solutions would
> not be imposed and the agency would not have an automatic
> right of entry to authorities.   (Hunter, D. 1983)

The next major issue raised by this study concerns the diversity of resources which health authorities, GPs and other health professionals should consider when planning services for health in pregnancy and early childhood. Recent reports on maternal and child health have clearly recognised that many of the major determinants of health are beyond the direct control of the NHS or the people working in it (see for instance the Court, Short and Black Reports and the Royal College of General Practitioners' *Healthier Children — Thinking Prevention.* This study has suggested ways in which health professionals working at the local level can develop closer links with agencies outside the NHS which may be able to make more direct interventions for promoting health. Planning for health is planning for social development — at both local and national levels — and we need to become more conscious of this priority. There is a vast repertoire of skills, knowledge and experience which can contribute to the delivery of preventive health care. There are also rapidly expanding technologies which should be harnessed: community broadcasting, local radio, television and telephones.

Those shaping health authority and general practitioner services should open their eyes to this wider vision of resources for health and find ways of working with them. Indeed, just as the NHS needs the expertise of epidemiologists, economists and statisticians, it seems it should also find a place for resource specialists who are experts in identifying and working with a wide range of different local agencies concerned with health. Such people would need special training and experience and might be drawn from the fields of community medicine, community nursing or health education. They would have more than a 'liaison' role, attempting to facilitate and support — and where appropriate co-ordinate — local resources for health. They would develop ways of disseminating information about promising innovations in the delivery of care. If the type of development agency described above is created, such a person would have a key role in working with it.

It is important that any such resource specialists have the status and professional acceptance to work with the family practitioner as well as the health authority services. The primary health care team, and GPs in particular, hold a crucial key to future developments in preventive health care. A few projects in this study have shown how GPs can develop their unique position for facilitating and supporting innovative experiments in delivering health care in the community. However, although a special search was made for such schemes coming from GPs, surprisingly few were found.

The explanation of this finding must be complex and probably reflects, to some extent, the strong influence of GPs' predominantly hospital- and disease-centred training. Perhaps part of the explanation lies also with their method of payment. GPs are not salaried employees but are self-employed, independent contractors. In the course of this study it became clear that some GPs may not embark on new preventive health care schemes unless they receive payment which will reimburse them for expenses incurred and the loss of their remunerative time. There is an urgent need for the government and GPs to find ways to overcome this problem: not necessarily with new monetary incentives, but by greater attention to the structure and organisation of primary health care.

The issue of advertising and canvassing for patients is also connected with the way in which general practitioners are paid. Part of a GP's remuneration is based on the number of patients on his or her list. It is considered unethical for GPs to advertise their practice or canvass in a way which may entice patients from other practices to join their own. Therefore some projects, particularly those involving general practices working with community groups outside the practice, may be discouraged. It seems therefore that the professional guidelines on advertising and canvassing in general practice may need to be reviewed to ensure that they do not inhibit these types of development.

There is an important rider to add to the study's observations about the variety of resources involved in delivering health care. The absence of schemes identified from the private commercial sector of health care has been striking. Perhaps this is because we somehow failed to find the relevant developments which may exist. It seems more likely, however, that it is due to our particular interest in ways of delivering preventive care to families with high health risks. Of course, if they have the resources, the private sector of health care will provide antenatal and pre-school health services to those who can afford them. But private medical care, unlike the NHS, is financed by its profits. There are few of these to be made in the business of preventive health care for the increasing numbers of families living in poverty and unemployment, or those who are homeless or live in depressed urban areas. For them the NHS, with its principle of equality of access for all, irrespective of income, remains a lifeline. If this is removed, there seems little chance that the private sector will replace it.

At first sight, it is perhaps surprising that so little information is available about relevant innovative experiments in the delivery of maternity and child health services. However the study has shown that the people who establish the type of schemes described rarely record the way in which they work. They often have no research experience and can give little time to evaluating the impact of their activities. Finding people with the interest, time and appropriate training to help with these tasks is a problem, particularly for community nurses and volunteers. Due to this lack of information those planning and managing the statutory services may have difficulty learning from such schemes and providing funding and support for them. There is a need — as recommended by the Royal Commission on the National Health Service (1979) — to find ways of remedying the acute shortage of trained researchers in the health service, particularly among the nursing professions.

Even if schemes are described and evaluated, the resulting information is of limited value if it is not made available to others. Many of the schemes in this study appear to be unknown outside their local area, some are not known even within it. There is an urgent need to develop more effective ways of disseminating information about ways of working in the community.

But our information gap will not be closed merely by recording and reporting. Those who hear information need to understand its relevance to their own situation. It appears that there is often a surprising lack of appreciation among health professionals about the potential of alternative ways of working; also about additional resources for health care coming from outside the NHS. Learning opportunities should be developed in health authorities, family practitioner services and in the training courses of health professionals, so that people can realise and gain confidence in the many different approaches applicable to health care in the community.

In this study I have been searching for the unusual and the successful: for schemes which show that the availability and acceptability of preventive services for health in pregnancy and early childhood *can* be improved. It is important, however, that these apparent success stories are read with their full implications. Delivering services to people who previously have not been fortunate enough to receive them exposes the relevant organisation — NHS, local authority or voluntary — to extra financial commitments in the short term, though perhaps saving money in the long term. Providing health care in difficult and stressful circumstances tends to be labour-intensive: remember the health visitors who identified previously 'unknown' homeless families and took them on to their case-loads. They were quickly overwhelmed by the extra work and additional health visitors were employed. At a time of severe cuts in public expenditure there is a danger that well-intentioned health authorities — and indeed, local authorities — will be forced to shut their eyes to the unmet needs of the parents and children who, because of their economic and social disadvantages, may be particularly vulnerable to ill-health, disability and premature death.

The incidence of families experiencing poverty and unemployment is continuing to increase. In terms of health, the primary preventive tasks must be concerned to reverse these trends and stop such situations from occurring.[1] Alongside such programmes there is an urgent need for the government to consider how it will maintain and develop the position of preventive health services for pregnancy and early childhood. It is hard to escape the conclusion that the community services, which have featured so prominently in this study, particularly those of health visiting and community midwifery, face a perilous future. In some areas of the country their staffing ratios are still well below the targets recommended by the DHSS. In addition, at the time of writing, health authorities are suffering severe and sudden cuts to their budgets which must threaten the very survival of some services. Within health authorities the power of the hospital sector in the competition for scarce resources is enormous compared with that of the community services. A strong case can be made for the provision of 'earmarked' development money for health authorities, specifically for preventive and community-based health schemes and for work attempting to reach the people with the greatest health risks.

In summary, the type of developments described in this book suggest that there is a large potential for improving the delivery of preventive health care in pregnancy and early childhood. It seems likely, however, that this potential will only be realised if there is sufficient investment in community-based preventive services by the government, health authorities and family practitioner services and relevant local authority departments. The potential for change will only be realised, also, if new ways are found to support and promote creativity in the planning and management of all services for health. Great imagination is needed if we are to mould our precious resources into new and more appropriate shapes for the health of families. The rights of parents and children to more active involvement in the planning of their health services will have to be recognised. All this implies that the training of health professionals should be modified so that they can form links rather than barriers between the resources, skills and knowledge of the many individuals and agencies which are concerned to promote health in the community.

Notes

1 A number of European countries have considerably more generous child, maternity and unemployment benefits and disability pensions than Britain.

References

Acheson Report: see London Health Planning Consortium (1981).

Adelstein, A.M., Macdonald Davies, I.M. and Weatherall, J.A.C. (1980) *Perinatal and Infant Mortality: Social and Biological Factors 1975—1977.* Studies on Medical and Population Subjects no. 41. HMSO.

Allen, R. and Purkis, A. (1983). *Health in the Round. Voluntary Action and Antenatal Services.* Bedford Square Press.

Ambler, M., Anderson, J., Black, M., Draper, P., Lewis, J., Moss, W. and Murrell, T. (1968). The Attachment of Local Health Authority Staff to General Practices. *The Medical Officer,* 295—9.

Aplin, G. and Pugh, G. (eds.)(1983). *Perspectives in Preschool Home Visiting.* National Children's Bureau and Community Education Development Centre.

Armstrong, G. and Brown, F. (1979). *Five Years On.* A follow-up study of the long term effects on parents and children of an early learning programme in the home. Available from Social Evaluation Unit, Dept of Social and Administrative Studies, University of Oxford.

Ashley, A. (1980). Voluntary Self Help for Parents under stress in Britain. *Midwife, Health Visitor and Community Nurse,* 244—6.

Association of County Councils (1979). *Rural Deprivation.* Available from Association of County Councils, 66a Eaton Square, London, SW1 W9BH.

Barclay Report: see National Institute for Social Work (1982).

Barnsley AHA (1978). Area Nursing Officers Report: Home Nursing and Health Visiting Services. Unpublished.

Barnsley AHA (1979). Home Nursing and Health Visiting Service. Area Nursing Officers Report. Unpublished.

Bayley, M., Parker P., Seyd, R. and Tennant, A. (1981). Neighbourhood Services Project, Dinnington. *Paper No. 1 Origins, Strategy and Proposed Evaluation.* Available from Dept of Sociological Studies, University of Sheffield.

Black Report: see Department of Health and Social Security, (1980) and Townsend, P. and Davidson, N. (1982).

Blaxter, M. (1981). *The Health of the Children.* Heinemann Educational Books.

Bogie, A. (1981). A Crying Baby Advisory Service. *Health Visitor,* 54, 535—7.

Boyd, C. and Sellers, L. (1982). *The British Way of Birth.* Pan.

Bradley, M. (1982). *Co-ordination of Services for Children Under Five.* NFER — Nelson.

Bradley, M. and Kucharski, R. (1977). *They Never Asked Us Before . . . Survey of Pre-School Needs in Liverpool.* Available from St Katherine's College, Liverpool.

Brent Community Health Council (1981). *Black People and the Health Service.* Available from Brent CHC, 16 High Street, London, NW10.

British Association of Social Workers Social Context Advisory Panel (1981). *The Cost of Caring: the Case for the Personal Social Services.* A Report. Available from BASW, 16, Kent Street, Birmingham, 5.

British Broadcasting Corporation Publicity and Information Department (1983). *Local Radio.* BBC Fact Sheet 27. BBC.

British Medical Association Council (1973). From Council. Police Bill Opposed. *British Medical Journal,* 286, 907—8.

Brown, G.W. and Davidson, S. (1978). Social class, psychiatric disorder of mother, and accidents to children. *Lancet,* 1, 378—80.

Brown, G.W. and Harris, T. (1978). *Social Origins of Depression. A Study*

of Psychiatric Disorder in Women. Tavistock Publications.
Bruce, N. (1980). *Teamwork for Preventive Care.* Research Studies Press. John Wiley & Sons Ltd.
Bruner, J.S. (1973). On Knowing. *Essays for the Left Hand.* Atheneum, New York. 12th edition.
Butler, N. and Alberman, E. (eds.) (1969). *Perinatal Problems: The Second Report of the 1958 British Perinatal Mortality Survey.* E. and S. Livingstone Ltd.
Butler, N., Golding, J., Dowling, S. and Howlett, B. (Forthcoming). *From Birth to Five.* Spastics International Medical Publications.
Calder, J. and Lilley, A. (1978a and b). *Self Help groups and the Role of Co-ordinators.* Nos. 1 and 2. Community Education Evaluation Group. Papers No. 2 and 3. The Open University.
Calder, J., Lilley, A., Williams, W. and Baines, S. (1979). *Informal and Alternative Uses of 'The First Years of Life' and 'The Pre-School Child' Course Materials.* Community Education Evaluation Group. Paper No. 7. The Open University.
Cambridge Community Health Council (1977). *Maternity Services.* Report of the survey of maternity services conducted March—June 1977. Available from Cambridge CHC, 21 Trumpington Street, Cambridge.
Cartwright, A. (1979). *The Dignity of Labour? A Study of Childbearing and Induction.* Tavistock Publications.
Central Advisory Council for Education (England) (1976). *Children and their Primary Schools.* HMSO.
Central Birmingham CHC (1981). *'6/10 Should Do Better'.* A Report on Parents' Perception of Child Health Services in Central Birmingham. Available from Central Birmingham CHC, 161 Corporation Street, Birmingham, B4 6PH.
Central Management Services (1982). *A Study of Interpreter Training Needs in the NHS.* DHSS.
Central Policy Review Staff (1975). *A Joint Framework for Social Policy.* HMSO.
Chaplin, N. (ed.) (1982). *The Hospital and Health Service Year Book 1982.* Institute of Health Service Administrators.
Chapman, S. and Reynolds, E. (1982). Postnatal Group for Mothers with Serious Mothering Problems. *Health Visitor,* 55, 461—6.
Childrens Committee (1980). Out-of-hours Social and Health Care. Report of a working group. *Health and Social Service Journal,* 90, CCI—CCII. 13.6.80.
Colley, J. and Reid, D. (1970). Urban and Social Class Origins of Childhood Bronchitis in England and Wales. *British Medical Journal,* 2, 213—17.
Committee of Enquiry into the Education of Handicapped Children and Young People (Chairwoman: Mrs H.M. Warnock) (1978). *Special Educational Needs.* Cmnd 7212. HMSO.
Committee on Child Health Services (Chairman: Professor D. Court) (1976). *Fit for the future.* Cmnd 6684. HMSO.
Committee on the Working of the Abortion Act (Chairwoman: The Hon. Mrs Justice Lane) (1974). *Report* Cmnd 5579. HMSO.
Commonwealth Health Ministers (1981). *Health and the Family.* Report of the 6th Commonwealth Health Ministers' Meeting, Arusha, Tanzania. 1980. Commonwealth Secretariat.
Community Service Volunteers (1981). *School Concern Project.* Final Report. Available from CSV, 273 Pentonville Road, London, N1.
Court Report: see Committee on Child Health Services.
Craven, R. and Breslin, S. (1981). Survey of the Telephone-In Service. Report of Survey of calls received at the Wrekin GP Maternity Unit

June—December 1981. Unpublished.
Davie, R., Butler, N. and Goldstein, H. (1972). *From Birth to Seven.* First Report of the National Child Development Study. Longmans.
Department of the Environment (1982). Biannual Count of Gypsy Caravans. Dept of the Environment.
Department of the Environment (1983). Gypsy sites provided by Local Authorities. Dept of the Environment.
Department of Health and Social Security (1976a). Joint Care Planning: Health and Local Authorities. HC(76)18./LAC(76)6. DHSS.
Department of Health and Social Security (1976b). *Prevention and health: everybody's business.* HMSO.
Department of Health and Social Security (1976c). *Priorities for Health and Personal Social Services in England: A Consultative Document.* HMSO.
Department of Health and Social Security (1976d). *Sharing Resources for Health in England.* Report of the Resource Allocation Working Party. HMSO.
Department of Health and Social Security (1977). Joint Care Planning: Health and Local Authorities. HC(77)17. DHSS.
Department of Health and Social Security (1980). *Inequalities and Health.* Report of a Research Working Group. DHSS.
Department of Health and Social Security (1981a). *Care in Action. A Handbook of Policies and Priorities for the Health and Personal Social Services in England.* HMSO.
Department of Health and Social Security (1981b). *Opportunities for Volunteering. A consultation paper by the Department of Health and Social Security.* DHSS.
Department of Health and Social Security (1981c). *Report of a Study on Community Care.* DHSS.
Department of Health and Social Security and Child Poverty Action Group (1978). *Reaching the Consumer in the Antenatal and Child Health Services.* Report of Conference 4.4.78. DHSS.
Department of Health and Social Security and Department of Education and Science (1976). Co-ordination of Local Authority Services for Children Under 5. LASSL (76) 5. DHSS.
Department of Health and Social Security and Department of Education and Science (1978). Co-ordination of Services for Children Under 5. LASSL (78) 1. DHSS.
Deakin, N. (1982). *A Voice for all Children.* Report of an Independent Enquiry. Bedford Square Press.
Denison, R.S. (1979). After Delivery Care. *Journal of the Royal College of General Practitioners,* 29, 499.
Douglas, J. and Blomfield, J. (1958). *Children Under Five.* Allen and Unwin Ltd.
Dowling, S. (1978). *Patterns of Contact Between Pre-School Children and their Services in the First Four Years of Life.* Unpublished. Thesis for Membership of the Faculty of Community Medicine.
Dowling, S. (1980). Services for the Health of Young Children and Their Families. Paper Given to the National Conference of BAECE, Sheffield. Unpublished.
Dowling, S. (1983). *A Question of Inter-Agency Collaboration for Family Health,* in White Franklin, A. (ed.) *Family Matters.* Pergamon Press.
Dowling, S. (Forthcoming). *The Provision of Community Antenatal Services,* in Zander, L. and Chamberlain, G. (eds.) *Pregnancy Care in the 1980s.* Macmillan.
Dunnell, K. and Dobbs, J. (1982). *Nurses Working in the Community.* OPCS Social Survey Division. HMSO.

Ealing, CHC (1978). *The Good Health Guide.* Available from Ealing CHC, 17 Churchfield Road, Ealing, W13.

England, H. (1980). Education for Co-operation in Health and Social Work. Papers from the Symposium on Interprofessional Learning, University of Nottingham, July 1979. *Occasional Paper 14. Journal of the Royal College of General Practitioners.*

Flack, G. (1977). Looking for dividends from the co-operative movement. *Health and Social Service Journal,* 432—5.

Fordham, P., Poulton, G. and Randle L. (1979). *Learning Networks in Adult Education.* Routledge & Kegan Paul.

Fraser, R. (1982). Patient movements and the accuracy of the age-sex register. *Journal of the Royal College of General Practitioners,* 32, 615—22.

Fraser, R. and Clayton, D. (1981). The accuracy of age-sex registers, practice medical records and family practitioner committee registers. *Journal of the Royal College of General Practitioners,* 31, 410—19.

Friend, J., Power, J., Yewlett, C. (1974). *Public Planning: the inter-corporate dimension.* Tavistock Publication.

Garcia, J. (1981). Findings on antenatal care from Community Health Council Surveys. Unpublished paper.

Garcia, J. (1982). *Women's Views of Antenatal Care,* in Enkin, M. and Chalmers, I. (eds.) *Effectiveness and Satisfaction in Antenatal Care.* Spastics International Medical Publications/Heinemann Medical Books.

Garcia, J. and Oakley, A. (1982). Is early antenatal attendance so important? *British Medical Journal,* 284, 1474.

Gath, A. (1978). *Down's Syndrome and The Family. The early years.* Academic Press

Gloag, D. (1983). A cooler look at lead. *British Medical Journal,* 286, 1458—9.

Gordon, P. (1980). *Good Practices in Mental Health. A guide to organising local studies.* Available from International Hospital Federation. 126 Albert Street, London, NW1 7NX.

Graham, H. and McKee, L. (1980). *The First Months of Motherhood.* Summary report of a survey of women's experiences of pregnancy, childbirth and the first six months after birth. Health Education Council Monograph no. 3.

Griffiths, K., Miller, P., Price, D., Flack, G. and Jameson, A. (1979). *Handbook of Exercises as an Aid to Multidisciplinary Training.* Available from E.N.B., Victory House, 170 Tottenham Court Road, London W1P 0HA.

Hadley, R. and McGrath, M. (eds.) (1980). *Going Local. Neighbourhood Social Services.* National Council for Voluntary Organisations. Occasional Paper One. Bedford Square Press.

Hall, M., Chng, P. and MacGillivray, I. (1980). Is Routine Antenatal Care Worthwhile? *Lancet,* ii, 78—80.

Hallett, C. and Stevenson, O. (1980). *Child Abuse: Aspects of Interprofessional Co-operation.* Studies in the Personal Social Serices no. 2. Allen and Unwin.

Ham, C. and McMahon, L. (1982). *The promotion of innovation in health care: the case for development agencies in the N.H.S.* A report of, and commentary on, a conference held at the Kings Fund Centre, 28.10.81. Kings Fund Centre/Royal Institute of Public Administration, London. Unpublished.

Hannam, C. (1980). *Parents and Mentally Handicapped Children.* 2nd edn. Penguin.

Harrington, C. (1981). An Evening on Call. *Health Visitor,* 54, 60.

Harrison, M. (1979) Home-Start. Report on its Development from November 1977 to March 1979. Unpublished.

Hatch, S. (1981). *The Voluntary Sector: A Larger Role?*, in Goldberg, E.M. and Hatch, S. (eds.) *A New Look at the Personal Social Services.* Discussion Paper No 4. Policy Studies Institute.

Haylock, M. (1981). A 24 Hour Health Visiting Service. *Health Visitor*, 54, 16—18.

Health and Safety Commission (1978). *Prevention and Health. Occupational Health Services. The way ahead.* HMSO.

Health Visitors' Association (1982). Inner London Health Care. *Health Visitor*, 55, 91.

Henley, A. (1979). *Asian Patients in Hospital and at Home.* King Edward's Hospital Fund for London.

Hevey, D. and Jackson, S. (1982). *Scope for Parents and Children.* A report on a utilisation-focused evaluation study. SSRC Preschool Evaluation Project. Unpublished.

Heward, J. and Clayton, D. (1980). The point accuracy of paediatric population registers. *Journal of the Royal College of General Practitioners*, 30, 412—16.

Hiskins, G. (1981). How Mothers Help Themselves. *Health Visitor*, 54, 108—11.

Homans, H. (1980). *Pregnant in Britain. A Sociological approach to Asian and British women's experiences.* Ph.D. thesis. Dept of Sociology, University of Warwick. Unpublished.

House of Commons Expenditure Committee (1977). *Preventive Medicine.* First Report. Session 1976—1977. HMSO.

House of Commons Hansard (1983a). 11.3.1983, 38, col 524W.

House of Commons Hansard (1983b). 19.4.1983, 41, col 76W.

House of Commons Home Affairs Committee (1981). *Report on Racial Disadvantage.* Vol. 1. Fifth Report. Session 1980—1981. HMSO.

House of Commons Social Services Committee (1980). *Perinatal and Neonatal Mortality.* Second Report. Session 1979—80. HMSO.

House of Commons Select Committee on Violence in the Family (1977). *Violence to Children.* First Report. Session 1976—77. HMSO.

Hubley, J. and Sheldon, H. (1980). *Health Education and Community Development.* A study of an area of multiple deprivation in the west of Scotland. Paisley College of Technology. Unpublished.

Humphries, B. (1976). *Only Connect. Lone parents and volunteers.* Available from Guild of Service, 21 Castle Street, Edinburgh.

Hunter, D. (1983). Promoting innovation in the NHS. *British Medical Journal*, 286, 736—8.

Independent Broadcasting Association (1981). *Independent Local Radio.* IBA.

Inner London Education Authority Educational Home Visiting Project, Deptford (1977). *Deptford Educational Home Visiting Project.* Research Report. Third Report. Available from ILEA, Central Offices, County Hall, SE1. 1977.

Inner London Education Authority. *S.E. London Educational Home Visiting Report.* Available from Joint Resource Centre, Frobisher Institute.

Jackson, B. (1982). *The Child Care Switchboard — An Experiment in using Communications to Help the Child at Risk.* The National Children's Centre, Huddersfield.

Jayne, E. (1976). *Research Report.* Inner London Education Authority Educational Home Visiting Project Deptford. ILEA. Unpublished.

Joint Working Group of the Standing Medical and the Standing Nursing and Midwifery Advisory Committees (1981). *The Primary Health Care Team.* DHSS.

Kensington, Chelsea and Westminster (South) CHC (1980). *'Maybe I Didn't Ask'.* Available from CHC, 89 Sydney Street, London, SW3 6NP.

Kidderminster CHC (1978). *'Is the baby all right?'* A Survey of Maternity Care in Kidderminster. Available from CHC, 184, Franche Road, Kidderminster.

Kings Fund Centre (1980). Health and Community Work: Some New Approaches. Available from Kings Fund, 126 Albert Street, London, NW1.
Kirklees Area Health Authority (1977). Huddersfield Health District Crying Baby Advisory/Relief Service. Report of Evaluation. Unpublished.
Knight, B. and Hayes, R. (1981). *Self Help in the Inner City*. London Voluntary Service Council.
Lancet (Editorial) (1977). The Abhorrence of Stillbirth. *Lancet*, i, 1188—90.
Lawrie, B. (1983). Travelling families in east London — adapting health visiting methods to a minority group. *Health Visitor*, 56, 26—8.
Lazar, F., Hubbel, V.R., Murray, H., Marilyn, R. and Royce, J. (1977). *The persistance of pre-school effects*. National Collaborative Study 14853. Available from Community Service Laboratory, Cornell University, Ithaca, New York.
Leat, D., Smolka, G. and Unell, J. (1981). *Voluntary and Statutory Collaboration*. Bedford Square Press.
Leicester, CHAR (1982). *Health Care for the Single Homeless*. Available from CHAR, 27 John Adam Street, London, WC4.
Lewis, E. (1982). Attendance for antenatal care. *British Medical Journal*, 284, 788.
Lilley, A. (1980). *The Local Radio Experiment*. Community Education Evaluation Group. Paper No 11. The Open University.
Linthwaite, P. and Sampson, K. (1983). *The Health of Travellers: Mothers and Children in East Anglia*. Save the Children Fund, 17 Grove Lane, Camberwell, London SE5.
London Health Planning Consortium: Primary Health Care Study Group (Chairman: E.D. Acheson) (1981). *Report on Primary Health Care in Inner London*. DHSS.
Lonsdale, S., Webb, A. and Briggs, T. (eds.) (1980). *Teamwork in the personal Social Services and Health Care. British and American Perspectives*. Croom Helm.
Maternity Alliance and Islington Community Health Council (1981). The Care of Pregnant Women at Work. Available from The Maternity Alliance, 309 Kentish Town Road, London, NW5 2TJ.
Maternity Services Advisory Committee (1982). *Maternity Care in Action. Part 1: Antenatal Care*. HMSO.
McAnarney, E.R. (1978). Adolescent pregnancy: a national priority. *American Journal of Diseases in Children*, 132, 125—6.
Merryweather, S. (1981). *English as a Second Language Teaching for Adults from Ethnic Minorities*. A NATESLA Survey Report. Available from NATESLA, Spring Grove Centre, Thornbury Road, Iselworth, Middlesex.
Ministry of Health (1954). National Health Service. Waiting Time in Hospital Out-Patient Departments. HM (54)52. Ministry of Health.
Morcroft, I. (1981). *The Milsom Road Project: Volunteers in Primary Health Care*. Available from The Volunteer Centre, 29 Lower Kings Road, Berkhamsted, Herts.
Moss, P. and Plewis, I. (1977). Mental Distress in mothers of pre-school children in Inner London. *Psychological Medicine*, 7, 641—52.
Mullen, P., Murray-Sykes, K., Kearns, W. (1981). *Survey of Planning Teams: Methodology and Basic Results*. University of Birmingham, Health Services Management Centre. Occasional Paper 29.
National Council for One Parent Families and the Community Development Trust (1979). *Pregnant at School*. Joint Working Party on Pregnant Schoolgirls and Schoolgirl Mothers. Available from National Council for One Parent Families, 255 Kentish Town Road, London NW5 2LX.
National Institute for Social Work (1982). *Social workers: their role and tasks*. Bedford Square Press.

Newell, K. (ed.) (1975). *Health By The People.* WHO, Geneva.
Norton, A. and Rogers, S. (1977). *Collaboration Between Health Authorities and Local Authorities.* Interim Report. Available from Institute of Local Government Studies, University of Birmingham.
Norton, A. and Rogers, S. (1981). *The Health Service and Local Government Services,* in McLachlan, G. (ed.) *Matters of Moment.* Nuffield Provincial Hospitals Trust. Oxford University Press.
Noyce, J., Snaith, A. and Trickey, A. (1974). Regional Variations in the Allocation of Financial Resources to the Community Health Services. *Lancet,* i, 554—7.
Nurses and Midwives Council (1976). *Pay and Conditions of Service.* Whitley Councils for the Health Services (Great Britain).
Office of Population Censuses and Surveys *Birth Statistics Series.* FM1 No 1 (published yearly). HMSO 1977—1980.
Office of Population Censuses and Surveys (1980). *Mortality Statistics. Childhood and Maternity. 1978. England and Wales.* HMSO.
Office of Population Censuses and Surveys (1981). General Household Survey. Preliminary Results for 1980. *OPCS Monitor GHS 81/1.* Government Statistical Service.
Office of Population Censuses and Surveys (1982a). General Household Survey. Preliminary Results for 1981. *OPCS Monitor GHS 82/1.* Government Statistical Service.
Office of Population Censuses and Surveys (1982b). Infant and perinatal mortality 1980. *OPCS Monitor DH3 82/3.* Government Statistical Service.
Office of Population Censuses and Surveys (1983a). Births by birthplace of mother 1981: Local authority areas. *OPCS Monitor FM1 83/3.* Government Statistical Service.
Office of Population Censuses and Surveys (1983b). General Household Survey. Cigarette Smoking: 1972—1982. *OPCS Monitor GHS 83/3.* Government Statistical Service.
Office of Population Censuses and Surveys. Social Survey Division (1983c). *General Household Survey 1981.* HMSO.
Office of Population Censuses and Surveys (1983d). Infant and perinatal mortality by birthweight: 1980 estimates. *OPCS Monitor DH3 83/1.* Government Statistical Service.
Office of Population Censuses and Surveys (1983e). Labour Force Survey 1981: country of birth and ethnic origin. *OPCS Monitor LFS83/1.* Government Statistical Service.
Osborn, A.F., Butler, N.R. and Morris, A.C. (Forthcoming). *The Social Life of Britain's Five-Year-Olds. A report of the Child Health and Education Study.* Routledge & Kegan Paul.
Oxfordshire CHC (1982). Where to Have Your Baby: the doctor gives the advice, YOU have the choice. Available from Oxfordshire CHC, 2 Market Street, Oxford.
Page, N.E. (1978). Community Experience in an Integrated Area. *Midwives Chronicle and Nursing Notes,* 81.
Paine, T. (1982). Survey of patient participation groups in the United Kingdom. *British Medical Journal,* 286, 768—72, 847—9.
Palfreeman, S. (1982). Mother and Toddler Groups among 'At Risk' Families. *Health Visitor,* 55, 455—9.
Parrick, M. (1979). 24 Hour Health Visiting Service or Crying Baby Service. Paper presented to Brent and Harrow AHA (Harrow Health District). Resources and Development Group meeting 24.4.79. Unpublished.
Peckham Health Project (1979). Report 1979. Pitt Street Settlement, East Surrey Grove, Peckham, London, SE15 5PP. Unpublished.
Plamping, D., Thorne, S., Gelbiev, S. (1980) Children as dental health edu-

cators. *British Dental Journal,* 149, 113—15.
Poulton, G. (1977). Reports on *The First, Second and Third Years of Scope, July 1976—79.* Unpublished.
Poulton, G. and Cousins, L. (1980). *The Fourth Year of Scope, July 1979—July 1980.* Unpublished.
Poulton, G. and Campbell, G. (1979). *Families with Young Children: A Hampshire-based Study Project.* Available from University of Southampton, Department of Education and Department of Sociology and Social Administration.
Pritchard, P. (1981). Patient Participation in General Practice. *Occasional Paper 17.* Royal College of General Practitioners.
Pugh, G. (ed.) (1980). *Preparation for Parenthood.* National Children's Bureau.
Reid, M.E. and McIlwaine, G.M. (1980). Consumer Opinion of a hospital antenatal clinic. *Social Science and Medicine,* 14A, 363—8.
Richman, N. (1976). Depression in Mothers of Pre-school Children. *Journal of Child Psychology and Psychiatry,* 17, 75—8.
Rimmer, L. and Popay, J. (1982). *Employment Trends and the Family.* Available from Study Commission on The Family, 3 Park Road, London, NW1 6XN.
Robinson, J. and Rosenthal, H. (1981). Having it Our Way. *Maternity Action,* 2, 11.
Rodmell, S. and Smart, L. (1982). *Pregnant At Work. The Experiences of Women in West London.* Open University/Kensington, Chelsea and Westminster AHA. Available from 304 Westbourne Grove, London, W11.
Rowbottom, R. and Hey, A. (1978). *Collaboration Between Health and Social Services,* in Jaques, E. (ed.) *Health Services.* Heinemann.
Royal College of General Practitioners (1982). *Healthier Children — Thinking Prevention.* Report of a Working Party appointed by the Council of the Royal College of General Practitioners. Report from General Practice 22. Royal College of General Practitioners.
Royal College of Obstetricians and Gynaecologists (1982). *Report of the RCOG Working Party on Antenatal and Intrapartum Care.* Available from RCOG, 27 Sussex Place, Regents Park, London, NW1 4RG.
Royal College of Obstetricians and Gynaecologists and The Population Investigation Committee (1948). *Maternity in Great Britain.* Oxford University Press.
Royal Commission on the National Health Service (1979) (Chairman: A. Merrison). *Report.* HMSO.
Rutter, M. (1966). *Children of sick parents: an environmental and psychiatric study.* Maudsley Monograph no. 16; Oxford University Press.
Sampson, K. and Stockford, D. (1979). Gypsy Children and Their Health Needs. Available from Save the Children Fund, 17 Grove Lane, Camberwell, London SE5.
Scarman, Lord L.G. (1981). *The Scarman Report. The Brixton Disorders 10—12 April 1981.* HMSO.
Scottish Health Education Unit (1980) *Book of the Child.* SHEU, Edinburgh.
Shields, J. (1979). *Report on Informal Interviews with Co-ordinators and Free Place Organisers for the Sponsored Places on P 911 'The First Years of Life'.* Community Education Evaluation Group. Paper no. 8. The Open University.
Short Report: see House of Commons Social Services Committee (1980).
Smith, C. (1982). *Community Based Health Initiatives.* Available from National Council for Voluntary Organisations, 26 Bedford Square, London WC1 B3HU.
Smith, G. (ed.) (1975). *Educational Priority Vol. 4: The West Riding EPA.* HMSO.

Smith, R. (1981). Health education by children for children. *British Medical Journal*, 283, 782—3.

Stockwell and Vauxhall Neighbourhood Council (1980). *Mawbey Brough: a Health Centre for the Community?* Available from Stockwell and Vauxhall Neighbourhood Council, 157 South Lambeth Road, London SW8.

Thornhill Neighbourhood Project (1982). *Antenatal Care: Who benefits?* Available from Thornhill Neighbourhood Project, 199 Caledonian Road, London, N1.

Towell, D. and Harries, C. (1979). Innovation in Patient Care: An Action Research Study of Change in a Psychiatric Hospital. Croom Helm.

Townsend, P. and Davidson, N. (1982). *Inequalities in Health. The Black Report.* Penguin.

Trades Union Congress (1981) *Women's Health At Risk.* A TUC workplace programme to improve the health of women. Available from TUC, London, WC18 3LS.

Trades Union Congress (1982) Collective Bargaining Agreements: Assistance for Working Parents. Unpublished.

Tudor Hart, J. (1971). The Inverse Care Law. *Lancet*, i, 405—12.

Unit for the Study of Health Policy (1979). *Rethinking Community Medicine.* Available from USHP, 8 Newcomen St, London SE1.

Van der Eyken, W. (1982). *Home-Start: A Four Year Evaluation.* Available from Home-Start Consultancy, 22 Princess Road West, Leicester.

Voluntary Organisations' Liaison Committee for Under Fives (1977). *Initial Discussion Paper* in Association of County Councils, Association of Metropolitan Authorities' *'Under Fives'. A Local Authority Associations Study.* Oyez Press Ltd, London.

Volunteer Centre (1976). *Volunteer Involvement in the National Health Service.* Evidence to The Royal Commission on The National Health Service. Available from The Volunteer Centre, 29 Lower Kings Road, Berkhamsted, Herts.

Volunteer Centre (1982). *Opportunities for Volunteering.* A response from the Volunteer Centre to the Department of Health and Social Security Consultation Paper. Available from The Volunteer Centre, 29 Lower Kings Road, Berkhampsted, Herts.

Wallis, S. (1977). *Bengali Families in Camden.* A report on the Community Health Project of Camden Committee for Community Relations. Available from Camden CCR, 335 Grays Inn Road, London, WC1X 8PX.

Walters, M. (1979). Postnatal Support. *Health Visitor*, 52, 416—19.

Wandsworth Council for Community Relations (1978). *Asians and the Health Service.* A Directory of Measures implemented by Area Health Authorities to Meet the Needs of the Asian Community. Commission for Racial Equality.

Wandsworth and East Merton Health District (1979). *Ethnic Minorities and the Health Service.* Report of the Working Party on the Provision of Health Services to Ethnic Minorities Living in the Wandsworth and East Merton District. Available from Wandsworth Health Authority, St Georges Hospital, Blackshaw Road, London SW1.

Warin, J.F. (1968). General Practitioners and Nursing Staff: a Complete Attachment Scheme in Retrospect and Prospect. *British Medical Journal*, 2, 41—5.

Warnock Report: see Committee of Enquiry into the Education of Handicapped Children and Young People. 1978.

Waterhouse, I. (1977). 'Dial-a-Midwife' — The Extension of Postnatal Care. *Midwives Chronicle and Nursing Notes*, 159—60.

Weatherall, J. (1982). A review of some effects of recent medical practices in reducing the numbers of children born with congenital abnormalities. *Health Trends*, 14, 85—8.

Weikart, D.P. and others (1978). *The Ypsilanti Preschool Curriculum Demonstration Project: Pre-school Years and Longitudinal Results.* Ypsilanti, Michigan: High/Scope.

Weissman, M., Paykel, E. and Klerman, G. (1972). The depressed woman as a mother. *Social Psychiatry,* 7, 98—108.

Werner, B. (1982). Recent trends in illegitimate births and extramarital conceptions. *Population Trends,* 30, 9—15.

West, R. and Lowe, C. (1976). Regional Variations in Need for and Provision and Use of Child Health Services in England and Wales. *British Medical Journal,* 2, 843—6.

Wightman, F. (1980). The Health Mobile. *Health Visitor,* 53, 422—3.

Williamson, J. (1980). *Self Help and the Doctor* in Hatch, S. (ed.) *Mutual Aid and Social and Health Care.* Association of Researchers in Voluntary Action and Community Involvement. Pamphlet no. 1. Bedford Square Press.

Wilson, A. (1977). Talking Point: Patient Participation in a Primary Care Unit. *British Medical Journal,* 1, 398.

Wiltshire Gypsy Council (1978). *A Special report on the health problems of Romany and Irish travellers in the South West, and Wiltshire in particular.* Available from Wiltshire Gypsy Council, 53 Longleaze, Wootton Bassett, Swindon. Unpublished.

Wolfenden Committee (1978). *The Future of Voluntary Organisations.* Croom Helm.

World Health Organisation (1981). *Global Strategy for Health for All by the Year 2000.* WHO, Geneva.